Schizophrenic Speech
Making Sense of Bathroots and
Ponds that Fall in Doorways

This book reviews our knowledge of the incoherent speech which is not uncommonly seen as a symptom of schizophrenia, and is one of the most researched symptoms in the disorder. The content covers clinical presentation, differential diagnosis and the theories proposed to account for the symptom of 'thought disorder', ranging from the psychoanalytic to there being a form of aphasia involved. The book is unique in its ability to apply linguistic and neuropsychological approaches, and is the first to cover comprehensively the range of clinical studies that followed the introduction of Andreasen's rating scale for thought, language and communication disorders. This book is essential reading for all those working in the field of schizophrenia and also for those interested in language and disorders of speech.

Peter McKenna is a psychiatrist with a special interest in schizophrenia. He has written one previous book on the subject and has carried out research, principally on the neuropsychology of the disorder.

Tomasina Oh strayed into the area of schizophrenic thought disorder during her PhD. A linguist by training, she is interested in language impairment, as well as the relationship between language and cognition.

Schizophrenic Speech

Making Sense of Bathroots and Ponds that Fall in Doorways

Peter J. McKenna

Consultant Psychiatrist, Fulbourn Hospital, Cambridge and
Visiting Professor of Psychology, University of Hertfordshire

Tomasina M. Oh

Assistant Professor, Department of English Language and
Literature, National University of Singapore

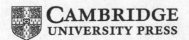
CAMBRIDGE
UNIVERSITY PRESS

CAMBRIDGE UNIVERSITY PRESS
Cambridge, New York, Melbourne, Madrid, Cape Town, Singapore, São Paulo

Cambridge University Press
The Edinburgh Building, Cambridge CB2 8RU, UK

Published in the United States of America by Cambridge University Press, New York

www.cambridge.org
Information on this title: www.cambridge.org/9780521810753

First published 2005
This digitally printed version 2008

A catalogue record for this publication is available from the British Library

ISBN 978-0-521-81075-3 hardback
ISBN 978-0-521-00905-8 paperback

The authors are indebted to two psychologists, Alan Baddeley and Rosaleen McCarthy, who over a considerable period of time influenced the writing of this book in many direct and indirect ways.

Contents

Preface

If ever there were a preface that ought to start with the words 'Why another book on ...', this is probably it. Thought disorder is the most studied symptom of a much-studied disorder, schizophrenia, and there has been a long tradition of punctuating the steady stream of publications on the subject with books. There may be some justification for continuing this tradition, in that the last single-author book on the topic was written in 1990, and, while there have been one or two multi-author volumes since then, it is fair to say that neither of these caught the tide of two major developments in the field. One of these was the wave of clinical studies that followed the introduction of Andreasen's rating scale for what she called thought, language and communication disorders; the second has been the rise of the neuropsychological approach to schizophrenia.

Naturally, neither of these developments was the reason for writing this particular book, which had more maculate origins. It grew out of our attempts to get a paper based on the research in a Ph.D. published. After engaging in the usual titanic struggle with the reviewers, one of us said to the other in a flash of exasperation that the only way we would ever get the damn thing into print was by writing a book on thought disorder and putting the paper in it somewhere. Immediately we both saw the possibilities for a book, and were quickly able to persuade ourselves that there was a pressing need for one, along the lines laid out in the preceding paragraph.

The phenomenon that forms the topic of this book has gone by many names over the years. Some of these have been picturesque and fanciful, such as word salad and knight's move thinking. Quite a few have come with their own theoretical baggage, either neurological, for example schizophasia, or psychological, as in the widely used American term, loosening of associations. Eventually, psychiatry settled on one of the most opaque terms ever used, formal thought disorder – the 'formal' denoting a disorder in the *form* of the thought processes as opposed to the disorder of *content* of thought exhibited by patients with delusions. As we wrote this book we grew more and more irritated by the clumsiness of this term, and its unintentional pretentiousness, and so we have substituted the simpler term thought disorder throughout. It may be more confusable with schizophrenic symptoms other than formal thought disorder, and purists may object that it excludes abnormalities of language (and communication), but it at least has the virtue of being less of a mouthful.

A number of people helped in the writing of this book in a number of ways. In addition to her general influence on our way of thinking, Roz McCarthy's knowledge of neuropsychology and aphasia was invaluable. We also owe her a debt of gratitude for patiently but determinedly persuading us that executive function might be relevant to some of the linguistic abnormalities of thought disorder, especially as one of us fought long and hard against accepting this. German Berrios informed the historical aspects of this book through his published work, many conversations and one journalistic interview; beyond this he also provided a great deal of deep background. The authors know a lot more about specific language impairment in children than they did before, after one of them spent an afternoon with Dorothy Bishop in Oxford. Statistically, Steve Graham and Raymond Salvador gave us a crash course in factor analysis, and Keith Laws taught us everything we know about meta-analysis. Paula McKay arranged a trip to Ireland to meet Senator David Norris in order to tap his extensive knowledge about James Joyce and his daughter, Lucia, and we would like to thank both of them for this. We are grateful to Cambridge University Press and Richard Marley for overlooking many missed deadlines. We would also like to thank Shirley Easton for battling to transcribe a number of indistinct recordings of often nearly unintelligible speech. Our families were incredibly tolerant with us, especially in the last few weeks before completion; we hope they know that their support was invaluable in the writing of this book.

Describing schizophrenic speech

When trying to explain thought disorder, or anything else for that matter, a good place to start is by describing the phenomenon accurately. In medicine, the customary way of doing this is by observing a suitably large number of patients who show the phenomenon in all its varied forms, and extracting the common features so as to arrive at some distillation of the essential nature of the symptom itself. This is the so-called clinical method, sometimes dignified as descriptive psychopathology in psychiatry, where the symptoms are much more individually variable than in the rest of medicine, and occasionally elevated to the status of its own discipline of 'phenomenology'.

Traditional and greatly respected in medicine, this approach to defining thought disorder was objected to by two linguists, Rochester and Martin (1979), on the grounds that it was too dependent on inference. They levelled their criticisms particularly at Bleuler (1911), who coined the term schizophrenia and was responsible for giving what is still one of the most detailed accounts of thought disorder. In the first place, he took it as a given that the underlying abnormality was one of thought rather than of speech, and according to Rochester and Martin the uncritical acceptance of this view by those who followed him caused many problems and obscured some interesting issues. Secondly, Bleuler specified the disorder of thought as one of 'loosening of associations' or 'association disturbance', a speculative construct to which he accorded great theoretical significance. But when Rochester and Martin turned to a contemporary textbook for a definition of loosening of associations they were confronted with statements like, 'In the loosening of association the flow of thought may seem haphazard, purposeless, illogical, confused, abrupt and bizarre' – which seemed merely to lead back to thought disorder. Clinical attempts to define the abnormalities contributing to thought disorder could, it appeared, all too easily descend into circularity.

Inferential and circular or not, observational studies have occupied a large part of the history of attempts to get to grips with what makes schizophrenic speech difficult to follow. One could begin an account of these attempts with Bleuler, Rochester and Martin's villain of the piece, whose sway was so great that his term loose associations became – and remains – a synonym for thought disorder. But, in fairness, this ought to be preceded by a description of the work of Bleuler's contemporary, Kraepelin, the originator of the concept of schizophrenia and a major influence on his and everyone else's views. Kraepelin's powers of observation are generally accepted as having been acute, and he had quite a lot to say about thought disorder, describing many of the phenomena in some of the terms that for better or worse are still in use today.

Kraepelin and Bleuler: the classical accounts of thought disorder

In his 1913 textbook, in which he gave his most detailed description of the symptoms of schizophrenia, Kraepelin (1913a) stated that 'the patient's mental associations often have that peculiarly bewildering incomprehensibility, which distinguishes them from other forms of confusion [and] constitutes the essential foundation of *incoherence of thought*' (italics in original). In less severe cases this showed itself merely as 'increased facility of distraction' and 'increased desultoriness', the patient 'passing without any connection from one subject to another', with an 'interweaving of superfluous phrases and incidental thoughts'. Sometimes, however, there could be an almost complete loss of connection between ideas. As an example of this he offered the following patient's reply to the question, 'Are you ill?'

You see as soon as the skull is smashed and one still has flowers [laughs] with difficulty, so it will not leak out constantly. I have a sort of silver bullet which held me by my leg, that one cannot jump in, where one wants, and that ends beautifully like the stars. Former service, then she puts it on her head and will soon be respectable, I say, O God, but one must have eyes. Sits himself and eats it. Quite excited, I was quite beside myself and say that therefore there should be meanness and there is a merry growth over. It was the stars. I, and that is also so curious, the nun consequently did not know me any more, I should come from M. because something always happens, a broken leg or something, they've had a quarrel with each other, the clergyman and she; a leg has just been broken. I believe that it is caused by this that such a misfortune happens, such a reparation for damages. I have also said I shall then come in the end last, with the sun and the moon, and too much excitement, and all that makes still a great deal of trouble. Kings do not collect the money, in this way the letters have been taken away from me, as I that at last of those that particularly believe as I at last specially think, and all are burned. You can imagine that comes always from one to the other.

Despite the on the whole completely aimless and fragmentary nature of the patient's utterances, Kraepelin observed that in a few places a certain connection between the ideas could still be made out, for example: *ill – skull smashed; held by my leg – not jump in; misfortune – reparation for damages; letters taken away – burned;* and *excited – quite beside myself.* This, he believed, pointed to an abnormality of thought ('it can scarcely be only a question of disorders of linguistic expression'). He used the term derailment[1] to describe this abnormality – a tendency for the line of thought to depart from the given idea and move in indistinct spheres of ideas. In some cases, although not in the above example, the deviation from one train of thought to another could be clearly identified. For example when asked what year it was, a patient replied 'It may be Australia', derailing from the series of years to the series of continents. The derailment could also be based on rhyme, a phenomenon otherwise known as clang association: thus a patient replied to a question about which town the hospital was in by saying, 'The house stands in the gospel of Luke of the eighth, and if one has swine, one can slaughter them' [German: *des achten . . . schlachten*].

At the same time, a disorder of language was also evident to Kraepelin. The above patient's syntax was confused in places, for example in *former service and then she does it*, and *I, and that is also so curious, therefore the nun consequently did not know me any more*, and *as I that at last of those that particularly believe*. Other patients showed a more severe disorder of grammar so that their speech became telegrammatic, doing without all superfluous phrases. Still others exhibited paraphasias and neologisms. The former took the form of a simple mutilation, change or partial fusion of commonly used words, or the substitution of one word with another, usually similar in sound or meaning, as for example in a patient who complained that his senses were 'checked'. Neologisms were new unintelligible words, which could be composed either of sensible component parts or senseless collections of syllables. To account for these apparent linguistic phenomena Kraepelin extended the concept of derailment to include derailment in the process of finding words.

Between thought and speech, Kraepelin felt he could isolate yet another form of derailment, this time in the expression of thought in speech (for which he introduced his own neologism, akataphasia). In this type of derailment patients used phrases or sentences where the words used only approximated to the thought that they wished to express. Thus a patient stated that he 'lived under protected police' instead of 'under the protection of police'; another said he had 'his fiancée always in speech' instead of 'his fiancée still continued to speak to him' (through voices).

If Kraepelin's only foray into inference and explanation was a somewhat awkward attempt to subsume several different elements of thought disorder under a single heading of derailment, Bleuler (1911) strayed much further into this territory. In fact, his book on schizophrenia was a tour de force of theory, which

---

[1] According to the historian of psychiatry, Berrios (personal communication), Kraepelin used a variety of German words in this connection, none of which was necessarily a railway metaphor. The English language term, which went on to become universal, was actually introduced by his translators, Barclay and Robertson.

began with a statement that certain symptoms were crucial for understanding the disorder by virtue of being 'present in every case and at every period of the illness even though, as with any other disease symptom, they must have attained a certain degree of intensity before they can be recognized with certainty'. First in his list of these so-called fundamental symptoms was association disturbance. As he put it:

> In this malady the associations lose their continuity. Of the thousands of associative threads which guide our thinking, this disease seems to interrupt, quite haphazardly, sometimes such single threads, sometimes a whole group, and sometimes even large segments of them. In this way thinking becomes illogical and even bizarre.

Loosening of associations led thinking to operate with ideas and concepts which had little or no connection with the main idea, and caused patients to lose themselves in irrelevant side associations. But alongside this Bleuler considered that there was another abnormal process at work, which was either closely related to the association disturbance or partly or wholly responsible for it (he never specified which). This was loss of the normal goal-directedness in thinking, a lack of the most important determinant of associations – that of purpose. In his words, 'thoughts are subordinated to some sort of general idea, but they are not related and directed by any unifying concept of purpose or goal.' He gave examples of patients who either wandered away from their initial topic of conversation or adhered loosely to it but covered a much larger group of ideas. Perhaps his most graphic example was a letter from a patient to his mother. After an unexceptional first paragraph the patient went on to write:

> I am writing on paper. The pen which I am using is from a factory called 'Perry & Co'. This factory is in England. I assume this. Behind the name of Perry Co. the city of London is inscribed; but not the city. The city of London is in England. I know this from my schooldays. Then, I always liked geography. My last teacher in that subject was Professor August A. He was a man with black eyes. I also like black eyes. There are also blue and gray eyes and other sorts, too. I have heard it said that snakes have green eyes. All people have eyes. There are some, too, who are blind. These blind people are led about by a boy. It must be very terrible not to be able to see. There are people who can't see and, in addition, can't hear. I know some who hear too much. One can hear too much. There are many sick people in Burgholzi; they are called patients. One of them I like a great deal. His name is E. Sch. He taught me that in Burgholzi there are many kinds, patients, inmates, attendants. Then there are some who are not here at all. They are all peculiar people . . . .

To Bleuler the letter demonstrated a complete absence of purpose – to convey to his mother how he felt, what made him comfortable or uncomfortable, or what might interest her. Otherwise, the chain of association could be considered perfectly valid: London – geography lesson – geography teacher – his black eyes – gray eyes – green snake-eyes – human eyes – blind people – their companions – horrible fate, etc. Nevertheless the letter was meaningless.

The combined influence of loosening of associations and loss of goal-directness of thinking enabled Bleuler to provide explanations for quite a number of different phenomena seen in thought-disordered schizophrenic speech. Hence, the partial interruption of normal logical associative processes meant that indirect associations and clang associations could gain control and direct the train of thought. Also, two ideas without any intrinsic relation to each other could become connected – for example a patient called a drawing of a comb a wash-tub because a wash-tub happened to be in the drawing next to it. For the same reason it was quite common for a reply to have nothing to do with the question posed: a patient was asked why she was not doing the household work she was supposed to be engaged in and replied, 'But I don't understand any French.' Instead of returning a greeting another said, 'That is the little Jew's clock in regard to Daniel.' Sometimes all the associative threads were broken, giving rise to complete blocking of thought, after which ideas could emerge which had no recognisable connection with preceding ones.

Bleuler recognised much the same range of disorders of word usage as Kraepelin – neologisms and use of words and phrases in an idiosyncratic way. He also accepted that the grammatical construction of sentences could be distorted. Besides the telegraphic style, he drew attention to an inclination to use convoluted sentence structures and pretentious and bombastic styles in both speech and writing; for example a patient wrote, 'The undersigned writer of these lines takes the liberty of sending you this by mail...'. But, just as Rochester and Martin stated, Bleuler seemed to go out of his way to avoid interpreting these as linguistic, invoking explanations in terms of thought whenever he could, and falling back on mechanisms involving catatonia, dreaming, etc., when he could not.

Cameron: the first empirical study of thought disorder

Cameron was an American psychiatrist who, with grant support of a distinctly unusual kind,[2] embarked on a study of thinking in schizophrenia, which was published in 1938. His original aim was to investigate parallels that authors like Piaget and Vygotsky had drawn between the reasoning of children and schizophrenic patients. However, his study soon metamorphosed into a descriptive account of thought disorder, but one in which the observations were collected under controlled conditions and recorded in a systematic way. Cameron's study is all the more interesting because he made it clear that he was approaching the field

---

[2] The Supreme Council, 33° Scottish Rite Masons of the Northern Jurisdiction, USA.

afresh, and in fact the conclusions he came to showed scant regard for the views of Kraepelin, Bleuler and other European authors.

The twenty-five patients Cameron selected for examination were diagnosed as 'quite unmistakeably schizophrenic' and they all showed 'scattering' at the time of examination, the term he used to describe thought disorder. Some were acutely ill patients at the prestigious Henry Phipps Clinic of the Johns Hopkins Hospital, whereas others were long-stay patients in the local asylum. To induce simple reasoning, he borrowed a technique from Piaget and gave the patients a series of uncompleted causal sentences, such as, *Your body makes a shadow because* . . . Replies were followed up by direct questions and requests for explanation. The investigator's questions and the patients' responses were recorded verbatim in shorthand.

From an analysis of this material Cameron picked out three factors that he considered made the patients' speech difficult to follow and which were distinct enough to justify separate discussion. These were: *asyndetic thinking, metonymic distortion,* and – introducing possibly the most eloquent term in the history of thought disorder – *interpenetration of themes.*

In asyndetic thinking, the substitution of loose clusters of terms for well-integrated concepts, the patient was unable to exercise the functions of selection, restriction and orderly arrangement necessary for the process of logical thinking, resulting in a striking paucity of genuinely causal links in speech. For example, when asked what makes the wind blow, one patient replied:

'Because it's time to blow.' [Question repeated] 'The air.' [The air?] 'The sky.' [How does the sky make it blow] 'Because it's high in the air.'

Cameron argued that this response consisted merely of a loose agglomeration of words connected with wind in general – wind, blow, air, sky, high (the initial reference to time was a perseveration from a previous answer). The patient clearly felt that the elements belonged together, but at the same time no genuine logical connection was present, even when the term 'because' was used.

This failure to bind together words and terms into an explicit explanatory construct was even more apparent in another patient's response to the same question:

[The wind blows] 'Due to velocity'. [question repeated] 'Due to loss of air, evaporation of water.' [What gives it the velocity] 'The contact of trees, of air in the trees.'

Here, Cameron pointed out, the elements of the response were not random, but consisted of phenomena which are commonly experienced directly or indirectly in connection with the wind blowing – velocity, loss of air, evaporation, contact with trees. Similarly, another patient answered the question:

[The wind blows] 'Because it howls.' [But why does it howl?] 'Lack of co-operation with the rain and the sun.'

Both responses were connected with the concept of wind, but only loosely: howling (physical feature) and rain and sun (other weather-related natural phenomena).

Cameron considered that a restriction of the patients' thinking to the matter in hand and even some degree of clarity of expression was impossible to miss, and there was surprisingly little real irrelevance. But, at the same time, there was an obvious lack of direction and no effective final pulling together of the elements into a well-formed whole. The patients' replies hovered around the problem rather than disposing of it. The material they produced was distant, too loose and too over-inclusive, a collection of fragments, a conglomerate not an integrate.

Metonymic distortion, or the use of word approximations, consisted of the substitution of a related term or phrase for the more precise definitive term that normal individuals would be expected to employ. Thus a patient said he was alive:

'Because you really live physically, because you have menu three times a day; that's the physical.' [What else is there besides the physical?] 'Then you are alive mostly to serve a work from the standpoint of methodical business.'

The most obvious word approximation here was *have menu* instead of 'eat' or 'have meals'. Cameron also felt *methodical business* was probably a distortion of 'daily routine'. In another example a patient explained why the sun comes up in the morning in the following way:

'Because it is the actual rotation of its axis between the arctic and antarctic zones.'

This substituted wide geographical areas for the more conventional terms, North and South poles.

Another patient considered that his body made a shadow:

'Because it hides the part of the light that is used for full room capacity or area capacity which you intervene.'

Here *intervene* was almost correct, but it should have been intercept. *Full room capacity* and *area capacity* both seemed to refer to the idea of complete illumination of a room and correctly implied the area from which the light is cut off by one's body, although the precise word or phrase was uncertain.

In other instances only a general sense of what the patient was trying to convey could be guessed at. Examples included: A fish can live in water . . . 'Because it's *the natural resource of life.*' A boy threw a stone at me . . . 'Because he had mischief and *arm exercise to exercise the body.*' I am good . . . 'Because brought up right and *strictly confidential.*'

Cameron felt that the use of these word approximations lent schizophrenic discourse a great deal of its peculiar elusiveness. It was as though the patient was using an idiom which could be translated into conventional usage, but which required effort to do so. As in asyndetic thinking, the words and phrases struck somewhere on the periphery of the target instead of the bullseye, and a false equivalence was attributed to several terms.

The material which became interwoven in interpenetration of the themes could be of fragments of different themes, or a theme and a counter-theme, but perhaps most typically one theme which was concerned with the immediate problem and another which reflected what Cameron called 'persistent preoccupations of a personal nature' – which by and large seemed to be delusions. He gave pride of place to the following example of a patient who had beliefs revolving around bodily injury, especially being bitten and having her back broken:

[A fish can live in water because . . .] 'Because it's learned to *swim*.' [What if it couldn't swim?] 'Not naturally, he couldn't. Why do certain gods have effects on *seas* like that? What does the *earth* have such an effect to break their backs? The *fishes* near home *come to the surface* and break.' [Why?] 'I think it is due to bodies that people lose. A body *becomes adapted to the air*. Think thoughts and break the *fishes*.'

The words and phrases in italics were vaguely relevant to the question put to the patient. Otherwise, sprinkled throughout her response were references to gods, bodies, back, effect, lose, break, etc., all of which reflected her usual delusional themes. Both lines of thought were equally represented, and were sometimes combined in to a single phrase, such as *The fishes near home come to the surface and break*, and *break the fishes*, and *a body becomes adapted to the air*.

In another example, a patient believed he was God and in a constant battle with the devil; he also constantly referred to 'the key to the outside':

[I get warm when I run because . . .] 'Because you possessing a position of a doctor have the key. The devil *seeing you run*, becomes ired. God doesn't get ired because it doesn't have any effect. He doesn't want a *railroad* or an *express company* in this place.'

The answer certainly incorporated elements of the question, as was evident in the italicised words, although phrases such as railroad and express company were only distantly related to the concept of running. However, the reply was mostly taken up by the battle between God and the devil.

The preoccupations did not have to be delusional. Cameron gave a further example of a patient who had unrealised ambitions to be an engineer.

[My hair is brown because . . .] 'Because it is a sort of hydraulic evering.' [What does that mean] 'It means that it gives you some sort of a *color-blindness* because it works through the *roots of the hair* and hydrasee – that is a study of the *growth of plants*, a sort of *human* barometer, hydraulic hydroscenic method.'

Hair colour was related correctly to roots of the hair and to growth. But the concept of colour was extended to colour-blindness, and growth to the growth of plants. In *human barometer*, the theme of the question and the theme of engineering appeared to be fused into a single impenetrable phrase.

Cameron argued that interpenetration of themes could be another manifestation of the same disorder of selection, elimination and focusing on the topic under discussion that was responsible for asyndetic thinking and metonymic distortion. In this case there was a failure of the normal process of subordination of one theme to another. Instead, elements of both proceeded together.

Cameron made several more minor observations. He noted that the patients were invariably fully satisfied with what were usually totally inadequate responses. Also, on the occasions they did give an initially fairly satisfactory answer, they often went on to add less relevant material; an initial good phrase would be followed by a jumble of peripheral concepts. Finally, he made the point that the abnormalities he found were potentially reversible and could improve markedly with general clinical improvement. He illustrated this with the patient's replies shown in Table 1.1.

Cameron's analysis was penetrating: again and again he managed to make sense of material that superficially could scarcely be more opaque. Some of the abnormalities he identified had counterparts in those previously described by Kraepelin and Bleuler. His asyndetic thinking embodied much of what these authors tried to capture with terms like derailment, loss of the central determining idea, and loose associations. Metonymic distortion was obviously similar to the abnormality Kraepelin referred to as akataphasia or derailment in the expression of thought in speech, although the specification was much more detailed and probably more accurate. In interpenetration of themes, however, he described a hitherto unrecognised clinical phenomenon, one which, as will be seen, was destined to have a chequered future career.

Table 1.1 Performance of a thought-disordered patient when severely ill and after partial recovery

(From Cameron, 1938)

During height of illness	After partial recovery
My hair is fair because . . .	
'Because of something else; it's on my head; it comes from my mother.'	'Because I inherited it from my parents.'
A man fell down in the street because . . .	
'Of the World War.'	'Because he slipped.'
The sun comes up in the morning . . .	
'Because it's a gas.'	'Because the earth goes around the sun.'
The wind blows because . . .	
'Just cosmic dust.'	'Because of atmospheric air-currents changing.'

Wing: poverty of content of speech

While carrying out a survey of male patients who had recently been discharged from long stay care in a mental hospital, Brown *et al.* (1958) made the surprising discovery that those with a diagnosis of schizophrenia were more likely to relapse if they went to live with their parents or wives than if they went to live with brothers and sisters or in lodgings. This was the starting point for a series of studies which established a major and still flourishing area of schizophrenia research, that of expressed emotion. It was also the point of origin for an abnormality that was to play an important part in the development of thinking about thought disorder, poverty of content of speech.

Wing, who joined Brown to work on two replications and extensions of his original study (Brown *et al.*, 1962; Brown *et al.*, 1972), had the task of interviewing recently discharged schizophrenic patients. For this purpose he was in the process of developing what would eventually become a widely used structured psychiatric interview, the Present State Examination (Wing *et al.*, 1974). During the course of the studies he came across an individual who showed a striking disorder of speech that he had not encountered before (Wing, personal communication). A sample of this, which was characteristic of all of the patient's conversation, went like this:

Q.   How do you like it in hospital?
A.   Well, er . . . not quite the same as, er . . . don't know quite how to say it. It isn't the same, being in hospital as, er . . . working. Er . . . the job isn't quite the same, er . . . very much the same but, of course, it isn't exactly the same.

Initially Wing was inclined to classify this a variant of poverty of speech, a symptom which was typically seen in withdrawn chronic schizophrenic patients. This symptom had been perhaps most eloquently described by Kraepelin (1913a) as the cessation of the need to express oneself:

The patients become monosyllabic, sparing of their words, speak hesitatingly, suddenly become mute, never relate anything on their own initiative, and let all answers be laboriously pressed out of them. They enter into no relations with other people, never begin a conversation with anyone, ask no questions, make no complaints, give their relatives no news.

Wing (1961) therefore incorporated this newly identified abnormality into the scale for poverty of speech. The maximal rating of 5 was made when the patient was mute or only spoke two or three words during the interview. A rating of 4 was given when the patient's answers were monosyllabic, often with long pauses or a failure to answer at all. A rating of 4 was now also given when 'although there was a reasonable amount of speech, the answers were so slow and hesitant, so vague and lacking in content, so repetitious and wandering, that meaningful conversation was almost impossible'.

The first full working draft of the Present State Examination (Wing *et al.*, 1967) had a section entitled 'Poverty of content, or restriction of quantity, of speech'. This had such items as, 'Patient is almost mute'; 'Patient frequently fails to answer'; and 'Answers are restricted to the minimum necessary'. There were also three items relating to poverty of content of speech. The first was 'poverty of content of speech', defined as: Patient uses quite a lot of words but says very little with them. No wandering from point to point. The second was 'vague wandering', with the definition: Patient talks a lot but meanders from one point to another, or circles round one point trying to express quite complicated ideas without being able to make his meaning clear. Brief replies to questions may be quite normal. The sentence structure (within the limits of conversational style) is not seriously distorted, and there is a serious attempt to convey meaning. The third item was not given a title, but was defined as: Longwinded, woolly, pedantic manner of speech with many redundant phrases, e.g. I believe we live in a world, in an age, where the elements are a force that the elders of professionalism hope, not to conquer, but to control.

By the final, published 9th edition of the Present State Examination (Wing *et al.*, 1974) this section had been reduced to a single item, poverty of content of speech. Wing *et al.* defined this as follows:

The subject talks freely but so vaguely that little information is provided in spite of the number of words used.

To which they added, not wholly tongue-in-cheek:

This symptom may appear to be readily recognizable in some of one's colleagues, therefore only rate it when it is really pathological.

Poverty of content of speech was now classified as one of three disorders of speech, whose effect was to make it difficult to grasp what the patient meant. The other two items were incoherence of speech and a form of thought disorder classically associated with mania rather than schizophrenia, flight of ideas. Neologisms were also included, but in another section.

Wing genuinely appeared to have identified a new abnormality of thought, which had been overlooked by earlier authors. If there were any prior descriptions, these were obscure. The only possible candidate is Kleist's (1930) term alogia. However, as described in Chapter 4, what Kleist meant by this term is far from clear. Wing also laid the foundations of a debate that continues to the present time: originally feeling that poverty of content of speech was more related to poverty of speech, he later changed his mind and decided that it belonged more with other disorders which made speech difficult to follow.

Harrow: thought disorder as bizarre-idiosyncratic thinking

Around the same time that Wing and his co-workers were developing their standardised mental state assessment, which became the Present State Examination, Harrow and co-workers (see Harrow and Quinlan, 1985) were carrying out an ambitious programme of research devoted solely to the symptom of thought disorder. Early on in this they concentrated their attention on the fashionable explanatory constructs of the day, including Bleuler's loose associations (e.g. Reilly et al., 1975; Siegel et al., 1976), concrete thinking (e.g. Harrow et al., 1974), the psychoanalytic concept of primitive drive-dominated thinking (e.g. Harrow et al., 1976), attentional disorder (e.g. Harrow et al., 1972a) and another cognitive disorder, overinclusive thinking, discussed in Chapter 7 (Harrow et al., 1972b). After a time, however, they came to the conclusion that a more descriptive approach might be in order: 'looking at disordered thinking in terms of more general concepts, such as bizarre-idiosyncratic thinking, is an alternate way of viewing it that can be quite productive'.

Harrow and his co-workers therefore began to explore bizarre-idiosyncratic thinking, a term they chose deliberately in order to reflect this new theoretically neutral approach to thought disorder. To this end they developed a standardised interview in which thought disorder was elicited by requiring patients to interpret proverbs like 'Strike while the iron is hot' and answer reasoning questions from the Comprehension subtest of the Weschler Adult Intelligence Scale (WAIS), such as, 'Why should we keep away from bad company?'. Bizarre-idiosyncratic responses were scored on a scale of 0 to 3 in various non-mutually exclusive categories, as shown in Box 1.1. All interviewers were trained with the assistance of a manual which defined and gave examples of the different abnormalities until they showed acceptable inter-rater reliability.

Box 1.1 Harrow *et al.*'s assessment of bizarre-idiosyncratic thinking

(From Harrow and Quinlan, 1985, reproduced with permission)

Responses to questions and proverbs are scored 0 – absent, .5 – minimal bizarre qualities, 1 – A definite idiosyncratic or bizarre response, 3 – A very severe bizarre response.

I Linguistic form and structure
A problem in this category implies that it is difficult to understand what the subject means owing to: (a) alterations in language, or (b) gaps in verbal communication.

Peculiar word form or use

Don't swap horses when crossing a stream. 'That's wish-bell. Double vision. It's like walking across a person's eye and reflecting personality. It works on you, like dying and going to the spiritual world, but landing in the Vella world.' [Comment: Neologisms are presented.]

Don't judge a book by its cover. 'A façade of regal compliance bides an aetiology of ire.' [Comment: Very pedantic – too abstract – out of proportion with the task.]

Lack of shared communication

The used key is always bright. 'The right path, you'll know the right path.' [Comment: The rater is impressed with a large amount of missing information. Very difficult to empathize with – little idea of where response comes from.]

II The content of the statement: the ideas expressed

This category pertains to peculiarities within a response that reflect confusion in ideas, peculiar or idiosyncratic logic, and asocial attitudes (descriptions of behaviour that most people would recognize as strange, unusual or taboo in our society).

Coherent but odd ideas

Why are people who are born deaf usually unable to talk? 'Because they have nothing to talk about except that they are bored.'

Deviant with respect to social convention

What would you do if while in the movies you were the first to see smoke and fire? 'I'd walk around in circles until I got dizzy and fell down asleep and dream about a passageway – wouldn't you?'

Peculiar reasoning or logic

One swallow doesn't make a summer. 'Summers are warm and it takes more than one summer to cool off.' [Comment: An illogical response. Also contains gaps in communication.]

Confused ideas

Why are people who are born deaf usually unable to talk? 'When you swallow in your throat like a key it comes out, but not a scissors. A robin, too, it means spring.' [Comment: Rater is impressed by lack of organization and coherence in the response. Verbalizations are generally confused and contradictory.]

III Intermixing tendencies

This category assesses tendencies to mix or blend material into the response from the subject's past or current experience, or to extend or elaborate a seemingly neutral theme or idea, making the response seem strange.

Box 1.1 (cont.)

The over-elaborated response

A rolling stone gathers no moss. 'That was a yesterday thing. If you keep yourself moving towards your goal whatever it may be and if you keep the goal in mind when you make decisions then you are most likely not to be led astray by feeling sorry for yourself, or greed or that type of thing. And if you just forget about your goals and values and give up hope and say the hell with everything, deteriorate, then you can get yourself in trouble.' [Comment: Here the amount of extra material is extensive. Also scored for intermingling.]

The intermingled response

A drowning man will clutch at a straw. 'Duh. Help! Is anyone going to save him. I could say I'm a drowning man right now. Anyone who asks for help. Ask and you shall receive. Seek and you shall find it. It all has to do with Christ.' [Comment: The answer is clearly affected by the subject's concern over his status and asking for help.]

IV The relation between question and response

The emphasis in this category is on determining if the subject is able to address the task of interpreting the proverb or responding to a question.

Attention to limited part of the stimulus

Don't swap horses when crossing a stream. 'Horses run courses, there are racetracks all over the country.'

The lack of a relation between the subject's statement and the question asked.

Why should we keep away from bad company? 'Say your prayers.' [Comment: There is little trace of the original question; the examiner has only a vague hint of where the response has come from.]

Why should people pay taxes? 'Show me the time to reason.' [Comment: Again it almost seems as if a different proverb or question is being answered.]

V Behavior

This category assesses behavior as it relates to conversational norms for conduct in a testing situation. A score in this category is attributed for behavior that is deviant, either in its extreme expression or in its incongruity and inappropriateness to the requirements of the situation.

What would you do if while in the movies you were the first to see smoke and fire? 'Report the fire (yells) FIRE! FIRE!' (runs around room wildly).

Using this rating instrument, Harrow's group were able to demonstrate that bizarre-idiosyncratic thinking was commonly but not universally present in acutely ill schizophrenic patients, lessened in prevalence and severity as clinical improvement took place, and became somewhat more marked again in the chronic phase of illness (see Harrow and Quinlan, 1985). Less prosaically, their assessment method led them to conclude that, while Bleuler's loose associations often seemed to be involved in the bizarre-idiosyncratic thinking of schizophrenia, this was not always the case, and in many patients bizarre verbalisations occurred without any noticeable looseness. Sometimes it was odd meanings and outlooks which made speech seem unusual. For example, a patient explained the proverb, *One swallow doesn't make a summer* as:

Just because a bird says it's summer and acts like it's summer, maybe it really isn't. Sometimes a bird could say it's summer, and it would really be winter.

Another factor Harrow and co-workers (Harrow and Prosen, 1978, 1979) identified in schizophrenic patients' bizarre-idiosyncratic speech was 'an intermingling into their verbalizations (and possibly into their thinking) of material that comes from their past or current experience'. How far they made this observation independently of Cameron's (1938) description of interpenetration of themes is uncertain, but in any event they did not acknowledge the similarity until several years later (Harrow *et al.*, 1983), and then only rather grudgingly.

Harrow's group appear to have been the first to draw attention to the fact that the pedantic or stilted speech in schizophrenia mentioned in passing by Bleuler (1911) could make speech difficult to understand in its own right (Harrow and Quinlan, 1985). One of their examples was:

Q.   Discretion is the better part of valour.
A.   Pliant rectitude is a trait more appropriate for successful living than hot-headedness which is either stubborn or crusady.

A further, longer and unwittingly poignant example of stiltedness, this time in a patient's writing, is given in Box 1.2.

Box 1.2 Stiltedness in a schizophrenic patient

The patient submitted the following document in support of his appeal against being detained in hospital:

Report re Hospital Managers Hearing
In address of: The Hospital Managers
From: Mr K– J–

Box 1.2 (cont.)

Introduction: Mr J– is vehemently objecting of slanderous reports bearant of his name submitted to the Hospital Managers and to associative means of appeal against legally enforced detentionable psychiatric treatment of his person.

Background: Mr J– is a forty-five year old bachelor who is a life-dedicated *yogi* which entails a lifelong commitment to maintaining the religious ordination and stipulates whereof his life is surrendered.

Mr J– is a former undergraduate of – University – whereof he has an open invitation to return to study having left volitionally in order to pursue a career in musical performing entertainment – and of – University which discharged Mr J– from a course of study in French and Italian in respect of a state of health determinantly unsuitable for the respective campus of the collegiate in 1979.

Mr J– actively attempted to achieve a personal ambition of full employment in a musical performancal entertainment until April 1989 – whereof a professional contract with Virgin Records was proffered – when he ended all personal association of musicianship owing to irreconcilable personal détente in professional life; since this time Mr J– whose musical compositions are known of the Royal Northern College of Music and whose name is *his* registered *copyright* has maintained a personal protestable denouncement of illegal utilisation of his song and musical work associated with a previous repertoire.

Mr J– is now a registered writer – having written a book of aphoristic poetry – and an oratorial (i.e. public lecturial) academic.

Mr J– is considered by his father, Mr R– J–, to be sufferant of the diagnosable disease of the human brain known in the medical term schizophrenic and has been recipient of this paternal party's adamant stratagem of implementing continuous psychiatric medical treatment thereof since he committed himself into the state of insanity after leaving the initiated life of devout religious yoga in the Indian Divine Light Mission* established in the United Kingdom of Great Britain and Northern Ireland in 1972 – being an alternative act to personal suicide.

Social 'History': Since a long touring holiday in 1993 Mr J– has lived in commercial board and lodgings in N– and surrounding region. He has been denied repeatedly the means of establishing his own home and has been able to maintain basic existence only in respect of Department of Social Security – and personal – attitudes and policies towards himself.

Signed

K– J–

* now known by the title ELAN VITAL, Reg'd Charity 24864

Harrow and co-workers' deconstruction and reconstruction of thought disorder ultimately took them in novel theoretical directions. They (Harrow and Prosen, 1978, 1979; see also Harrow and Miller, 1980) speculated that intermingling or interpenetration of themes, which implied an inability to prevent one's own internal context from intruding into speech, might be due to a failure to monitor and edit personal material out of speech, and that this in turn pointed to failure in 'specific aspects of the executive function . . . involved in controlling and guiding language and behavior'. They also raised the possibility that this and other features of thought disorder might involve what they termed impaired perspective, a general impairment of social knowledge and understanding of social conventions relating to speech and discourse. Both of these ideas subsequently went on to become important topics in thought disorder research and are discussed at length in Chapters 5 and 6.

Andreasen: the modern synthesis

In the 1970s American psychiatry was in crisis. This was the final chapter in what had been an almost complete takeover of mainstream psychiatry by psychoanalysis in this country. As recounted by Shorter (1997) in his history of 20th century psychiatry, in the heyday of this movement in the 1950s and 1960s virtually every prestigious chair of psychiatry in America was occupied by a psychoanalyst. Analysts and analysis sympathisers had taken over much of the apparatus of the American Psychiatric Association. Analysts wrote the textbooks, staffed the university departments and sat on the examination boards. Analysts were consulted by government agencies and Congress. Psychoanalysis was the basic science of psychiatry.

Central to psychoanalysis was the belief that symptoms were only symbols of underlying psychological traumas and conflicts, and diagnosis was a sterile exercises which only served to distract the clinician from the all-important underlying problems. Influential figures like Menninger and Meyer[3] proposed that all forms of mental illness were qualitatively the same, with schizophrenia merely being the most severe end of a continuum of pathological adaptations to the environment.

What followed, predictably, was a succession of high-profile diagnostic embarrassments, almost all of which revolved around schizophrenia. A particularly notorious example was when an international collaborative study (Cooper et al., 1972)

---

[3] The pre-eminent American psychiatrist of his day, who was also the director of the institute where Cameron worked and suggested the idea for his study. Meyer rejected the standard classification of psychiatric disorders and replaced it with a system of 'reaction types', such as anergasia, dysergasia, thymergasia and parergasia, which, probably to everyone's relief, failed to catch on.

was set up to investigate why the rates of diagnosis of schizophrenia and mania differed in Britain and America by up to ten- or twenty-fold in some age groups. The investigators expected to find that at least some of the variation would be due to genuine differences in the presentations of psychiatric illness in the two countries. Instead it quickly became clear that the differences were almost entirely a function of the American concept of schizophrenia, which was being applied to patients who, in the rest of the world, would be diagnosed as suffering from mania, depression, neurosis and personality disorder.

It was this disregard of diagnosis which led to the downfall of American psychodynamic psychiatry. How this came about – in what was to all intents a palace coup within the American Psychiatric Association – has been reconstructed by Wilson (1993) in one of the very few psychiatric articles that can be described as making gripping reading (see Box 1.3). As in many revolutions, a book – or in this case a manual – played an important role: the third edition of the Diagnostic and Statistical Manual, or DSM III. Previously a short reference guide to psychiatric diagnostic categories, the main use of which was for the compilation of official statistics, this became a psychiatric textbook in all but name, featuring sections devoted to the prevalence, age and sex distribution, course, familial pattern, laboratory findings and differential diagnosis of each disorder. DSM III laid down precise clinical guidelines for every diagnosis, from schizophrenia to premature ejaculation, and these depended on the presence of certain symptoms as defined in a glossary, in certain combinations, with certain exclusions, for certain periods of time.

Providing clear and unambiguous definitions of symptoms like delusions and hallucinations for DSM III presented few problems; all that was required was to describe the phenomenon clearly, indicate any similar symptoms it could be confused with, and perhaps give some examples. In the case of thought disorder, however, the difficulties were more serious. Not only did a set of symptoms have to be selected from what was by now a quite large and overlapping body of descriptive terms, each of these had to be defined in a way that allowed them to be used with an acceptable degree of reliability.

Andreasen (1979a), a psychiatrist who had previously published a number of papers on thought disorder, took on the job of developing and evaluating such a set of definitions. These were to be incorporated in the glossary of DSM III, and so, it was hoped, would become standard for American psychiatry. As a first step, she generated a deliberately inclusive set of terms. Her approach was strictly descriptive: the definitions 'were written to describe speech and language disorders commonly encountered in psychiatric patients without any attempt to characterise underlying cognitive processes'. Loose associations was an immediate casualty, excluded ostensibly because it was based on an outdated associationist psychology, but almost certainly also because American psychodynamic

Box 1.3 DSM III and the transformation of American Psychiatry

(From Wilson, 1993)

By the late 1960s American psychodynamic psychiatry was under attack on several fronts. In addition to embarrassing revelations about poor diagnostic practice, little if any meaningful research was being carried out and medications such as antidepressants, lithium and neuroleptics were proving to be effective. Another major factor was that both the government and private insurance companies were increasingly perceiving psychiatry as a voracious consumer of dollars with little transparency about what services were being provided and why.

   In 1974, the American Psychiatric Association created a task force to revise their 134-page diagnostic and statistical manual, DSM II. They were obliged to do this because of a treaty between America and the World Health Organisation, which was updating its own International Classification of Diseases. The individual chosen to head this task force was Spitzer. The focus of his academic career had been the development of various structured interviews for psychiatric assessment, and he had led a group which developed the Research Diagnostic Criteria, a symptom-based and rule-driven method of making diagnoses for research purposes. This group had rejected the psychodynamic model because it did not lend itself to reliable diagnosis.

   At first, the development of another diagnostic manual held little interest for psychodynamically oriented psychiatrists. However, a clinician on the task force soon expressed concern that the narrow definitions of syndromes being developed would mean that many patients who were currently in therapy would be said to have no disorder. Spitzer rebutted this criticism, on the grounds that insurance reimbursement would be difficult if the symptom clusters in the manual were not called syndromes, and research would be difficult without proper diagnostic categories. Later, a psychoanalyst who was added to the committee after it was set up resigned because he felt his suggestions had been dismissed out of hand. As the realisation grew that something very important was being done by a small group of psychiatrists, the American Psychiatric Association created a second committee to try and control the first.

   Despite continuing protests and the re-instatement of the term neurosis, which had been removed at an early stage, as 'neurotic disorder', DSM III was published in 1980. Its preface described the event as being met by 'interest, alarm, despair, excitement and joy'. Other reactions ranged from its being described as 'a fateful point in the history of the American psychiatric profession', to 'the emperor's new clothes'.

psychiatry had elevated Bleuler's (1911) statement that association disturbance was present in every case and at every period of illness to the level of incontrovertible truth. Instead she substituted the more descriptive and atheoretical term, derailment. She also re-introduced four additional terms that had previously been subsumed under loosening of associations – tangentiality, incoherence, illogicality and clanging.

There was no attempt to restrict the set of abnormalities only to those traditionally associated with schizophrenia. DSM III covered all psychiatric disorders, and, in any case, clinical experience suggested that some abnormalities classically associated with schizophrenia could also occur in other psychiatric disorders, such as mania and depression. Also, recalling Wing's observation about poverty of content of speech, there was good reason to suppose that some abnormalities would be encountered in individuals without a psychotic diagnosis.

In arriving at the final choice of terms, Andreasen also made a number of decisions to redefine, combine or delete older concepts in the interest of enhancing reliability. Thus, while the term tangentiality was retained, it was partially redefined to refer only to oblique answers to questions and not to transitions in a passage of speech. Rather more ruthlessly, flight of ideas, probably the most widely used term to describe thought disorder associated with mania, was dropped. This was on the grounds that 'it is probably impossible to achieve good reliability when clinicians must make judgments on how close relationships are between various ideas'. The phenomenon was instead parcelled out under the headings of derailment and pressure of speech.

The initial selection process resulted in a set of eighteen disorders of thought, language and communication, which are summarised in Box 1.4. The list was on the whole uncontroversial and most of the descriptive terms proposed over the last century survived to make an appearance. Some items, such as illogicality and stilted speech, were for the first time placed on an equal footing with the major abnormalities like derailment and distractible speech. All the definitions were explicit, and in some cases were an order of magnitude more precise and prescriptive than anything previously seen. For example, the abnormality in incoherence was specified as occurring within sentences themselves, as distinct from derailment where the lack of connection was between successive sentences or ideas.

The only surprising omission was interpenetration of themes. There was, however, an abnormality termed self-reference, for which the following example was given:

Interviewer. What time is it?

Patient. Seven o'clock. That's my problem. I never know what time it is. Maybe
    I should try to keep better track of the time.

While not similar to anything Cameron (1938) described, this was reminiscent of some of the examples Harrow and Quinlan (1985) gave of intermingling, for

---

Box 1.4 Abnormalities of thought, language and communication

(From Andreasen, 1979a, reproduced with permission from Archives of General Psychiatry, **36**, 1315–1321, copyright-© 1979, American Medical Association)

Poverty of speech (poverty of thought, laconic speech)
Restriction in the amount of spontaneous speech, so that replies to questions tend to be brief, concrete and unelaborated. Unprompted additional information is rarely provided. Replies may be monosyllabic, and some questions may be left unanswered altogether. When confronted with this speech pattern, the interviewer may find himself frequently prompting the patient to encourage elaboration of replies.

Poverty of content of speech (poverty of thought, empty speech, alogia, verbigeration)
Although replies are long enough so that speech is adequate in amount, it conveys little information. Language tends to be vague, often over-abstract or over-concrete, repetitive and stereotyped. The interviewer may recognise this finding by observing that the patient has spoken at some length, but has not given adequate information to answer the question. Alternatively, the patient may provide enough information to answer the question, but require many words to do so, so that a lengthy reply can be summarised in a sentence or two. Sometimes the interviewer may characterise the speech as 'empty philosophizing'.

Pressure of speech
An increase in the amount of spontaneous speech as compared with what is considered ordinary or socially customary. The patient talks rapidly and is difficult to interrupt. Some sentences may be left uncompleted because of eagerness to get on to a new idea. Simple questions that could be answered in only a few words or sentences will be answered at great length, so that the answer takes minutes rather than seconds, and indeed may not stop at all if the speaker is not interrupted. Even when interrupted, the speaker often continues to talk. Speech tends to be loud and emphatic. Sometimes speakers with severe pressure will talk without any social stimulation, and talk even though no one is listening.

Distractible speech
During the course of a discussion or interview, the patient repeatedly stops talking in the middle of a sentence or idea and changes the subject in response to a nearby stimulus, such as an object on a desk, the interviewer's clothing or appearance, etc.

Box 1.4 (cont.)

Tangentiality

Replying to a question in an oblique, tangential or even irrelevant manner. The reply may be related to the question in some distant way. Or the reply may be unrelated and seem totally irrelevant. In the past, tangentiality has been used as roughly equivalent to loose associations or derailment. The concept of tangentiality has been partially redefined so that it refers only to questions and not to transitions in spontaneous speech.

Derailment (loose associations, flight of ideas)

A pattern of spontaneous speech in which the ideas slip off the track on to another one that is clearly but obliquely related, or on to one that is completely unrelated. Things may be said in juxtaposition that lack a meaningful relationship, or the patient may shift idiosyncratically from one frame of reference to another. At times, there may be a vague connection between the ideas; at others, none will be apparent. Perhaps the commonest manifestation of this disorder is a slow, steady slippage, with no single derailment being particularly severe, so that the speaker gets farther and farther off the track with each derailment, without showing any awareness that his reply no longer has any connection with the question that was asked.

Incoherence (word salad, schizophasia, paragrammatism)

A pattern of speech that is essentially incomprehensible at times. The incoherence is due to several different mechanisms, which may sometimes all occur simultaneously. Sometimes the rules of grammar and syntax are ignored, and a series of words or phrases seem to be joined together arbitrarily and at random. Sometimes the disturbance appears to be at a semantic level, so that words are substituted in a phrase or sentence so that the meaning seems to be distorted or destroyed. Sometimes 'cementing words' (conjunctions such as 'and' and 'although' and adjectival pronouns such as 'the', 'a' and 'an') are deleted. Sometimes portions of coherent sentences may be observed in the midst of a sentence that is incoherent as a whole.

Illogicality

A pattern of speech in which conclusions are reached that do not follow logically. This may take the form of non sequiturs, in which the patient makes a logical inference between two clauses that is unwarranted or illogical. It may take the form of faulty inductive inferences. It may also take the form of reaching conclusions based on faulty premises without any actual delusional thinking.

Clanging

A pattern of speech in which sounds rather than meaningful relationships appear to govern word choice, so that the intelligibility of the speech is impaired and redundant words are introduced. In addition to rhyming relationships, this pattern of speech may also include punning associations, so that a word similar in sound brings in a new thought.

Neologisms

New word formations. A neologism is defined here as a completely new word or phrase whose derivation cannot be understood. Sometimes the term 'neologism' has also been used to mean a word that has been incorrectly built up but with origins that are understandable as due to a misuse of the accepted methods of word formation. For purposes of clarity, these should he referred to as word approximations.

Word approximations (paraphasia, metonyms)

Old words that are used in a new and unconventional way, or new words that are developed by conventional rules of word formation. Often the meaning will be evident even though the usage seems peculiar or bizarre (i.e., gloves referred to as 'handshoes', a ballpoint pen referred to as a 'paperskate', etc.). Sometimes the word approximations may be based on the use of stock words, so that the patient uses one or several words repeatedly in ways that give them a new meaning (i.e., a watch may be called a 'time vessel', the stomach a 'food vessel', a television set a 'news vessel', etc.).

Circumstantiality

A pattern of speech that is very indirect and delayed in reaching its goal idea. In the process of explaining something, the speaker brings in many tedious details and sometimes makes parenthetical remarks. Circumstantial replies or statements may last for many minutes if the speaker is not interrupted and urged to get to the point. Interviewers will often recognise circumstantiality on the basis of needing to interrupt the speaker to complete the process of history taking within an allotted time.

Loss of goal

Failure to follow a chain of thought through to its natural conclusion. This is usually manifested in speech that begins with a particular subject wanders away from the subject and never returns to it. The patient may or may not be aware that he has lost his goal. This often occurs in association with derailment.

Perseveration

Persistent repetition of words, ideas or subjects, so that once a patient begins a particular subject or uses a particular word, he continually returns to it in the process of speaking.

Box 1.4 (cont.)

Echolalia
A pattern of speech in which the patient echoes words or phrases of the inter-viewer. Typical echolalia tends to be repetitive and persistent. The echo is often uttered with a mocking, mumbling or staccato intonation.

Blocking
Interruption of a train of speech before a thought or idea has been completed. After a period of silence lasting from a few seconds to minutes, the person indicates that he cannot recall what he had been saying or meant to say. Blocking should only be judged to be present if a person voluntarily describes losing his thought or if on questioning by the interviewer he indicates that that was his reason for pausing.

Stilted speech
Speech that has an excessively formal quality. It may seem rather quaint or outdated, or may appear pompous, distant or over polite. The stilted quality is usually achieved through use of particular word choices (multisyllabic when monosyllabic alterna-tives are available and equally appropriate), extremely polite phraseology ('Excuse me madam, may I request a conference in your office at your convenience'), or stiff and formal syntax ('Whereas the attorney comported himself indecorously, the physician behaved as is customary for a born gentleman').

Self-reference
A disorder in which the patient repeatedly refers the subject under discussion back to himself when someone else is talking and also refers apparently neutral subjects to himself when he himself is talking.

instance that in Box 1.2. Self-reference may, therefore, have been the result of another of Andreasen's exercises in combination and redefinition. Whether it lost something in translation as a result is a moot point.

Three items reflected Andreasen's stated aim of being inclusive: poverty of speech, echolalia and perseveration. Poverty of speech does not in itself make speech difficult to follow. Echolalia is a catatonic symptom. Perseveration, the persistent repetition of words, ideas or subjects, so that once a patient begins a particular subject or uses a particular word he continually returns to it, is well-described in schizophrenia, but not particularly in thought-disordered schizo-phrenia, and is also characteristic of neurological disorders affecting cognitive function, especially dementia and the frontal lobe syndrome.

One item, circumstantiality, was described as being very common in non-patients, a reference to the familiar long-windedness of certain individuals. Andreasen differentiated this abnormality from poverty of content of speech in that the subject provided a wealth of amplifying or illustrative detail, and from derailment and loss of goal by the fact that the details presented were closely related to some particular idea and that goal was eventually reached.

Andreasen (1979a) then tested the inter-rater reliability of the 18 items she had isolated. For this, the abnormalities were rated on a scale of 0 (absent) to 4 or 5 (severe). A pilot study on a mixed group of forty-four patients with schizophrenia, mania and depression indicated that agreement was sufficiently good to continue, and after minor revisions the scale was used to assess the speech of sixty-nine further similar patients. Two raters conducted a forty-five-minute interview in which the patient was first invited to talk without interruption for about ten minutes. After this open-ended questions were asked, ranging from 'How far did you go in school?' and 'What do you think of President Nixon?' to 'Why do people believe in God?' and 'Tell me about your first sexual experience.' There were no questions concerning symptoms and so it was possible for the interviewers to remain blind to diagnosis. Of the eighteen definitions, only six were found to have weighted kappa values of less than 0.6, a figure commonly used as a cutoff for good reliability. These were tangentiality, clanging and echolalia, which fell just below the threshold; plus self-reference and neologisms, which were more substantially below it; and word approximations, which showed very low reliability. However, Andreasen noted that with the exception of tangentiality, which was the most marginal failure, these items were only rated very infrequently, making the kappa values inaccurate due to lack of variance.

Conclusion

Most of Andreasen's elements of thought disorder did find their way into the glossary of DSM III, although also included were loose associations and flight of ideas. Her Thought Language and Communication (TLC) scale, as it became known, went on to become standard anyway, and has been employed in nearly all contemporary studies of thought disorder. The final set of abnormalities, which she arrived at by her method of combining, redefining and deleting, has become only slightly less widely accepted as definitive. While most of these can be reliably identified, and so go some way to meeting the objections raised by Rochester and Martin, the altogether trickier question of their validity – whether the way in which they capture the phenomena of thought disorder is intrinsically meaningful – remains unanswered. This is the subject of the next chapter.

2

Thought disorder as a syndrome in schizophrenia

If the descriptive psychopathological or phenomenological approach to classification is to be believed, what clinicians lump together as thought disorder is really a disparate group of abnormalities, most of which can make speech difficult to follow on their own, but which are prone to occur in combination. Some of these abnormalities appear to lie in the realm of thought, some in the realm of language, and some in whatever is bracketed by these two concepts. Others may be mirror images of each other or even polar opposites, for example poverty of speech and pressure of speech. Still others just do not seem to be particularly closely related to each other – whatever it is that gives rise to derailment does not seem intuitively likely to be the same as what underlies, say, stilted speech or self-reference.

The set of abnormalities in Andreasen's TLC scale can claim some legitimacy by virtue of being the survivors of a process of natural selection, which saw several alleged phenomena simply die out. It is also true that they can be identified reliably. Even so, the range of abnormalities remains embarrassingly large, and reliability is no guarantee of validity. It may be that a century of deliberation has led to an accurate and complete taxonomy of thought disorder. But it could also be true that the modern classification of thought disorder is nothing more than an example of psychiatry doing what it is regularly accused of doing, namely applying labels to psychological phenomena in an artificial way which obscures their real underlying relationships.

This problem is not unique to thought disorder. Ultimately, there is no way of knowing whether the way psychiatry identifies any of its symptoms is valid, because there is no objective yardstick to judge them against. What can be done – and what psychiatry and psychology have devoted a great deal of effort to doing – is to examine the relationships among symptoms statistically. This approach has had a certain amount of success with broad diagnostic questions, for example whether there are one, two, or more distinct forms of depression, and how far the clinical features of schizophrenia and manic-depressive psychosis differ from each other. By chance, the application of statistics to a further much-researched question, of whether there are subdivisions within schizophrenia itself, has turned out to have an important bearing on thought disorder as a clinical concept.

The same methods can be, and in a limited way have been, applied to the individual symptoms that make up thought disorder, in order to determine whether it has a deep structure and if so what this is.

Subdividing schizophrenia I: subtypes of patients

It is a truism to state that schizophrenia is a heterogeneous disorder. The term encompasses a vast array of symptoms, which combine and recombine in an endless variety of ways in different patients, and in the same patient at different times. The illness follows many different courses, from single, self-limiting attacks, through relapses and remissions, to a slow, steady deterioration. The ultimate outcome can be anything from complete recovery to profound permanent disability. Even those who firmly believe that schizophrenia is a single disease entity often find themselves wishing it could be broken down into some more homogeneous subunits.

The first attempt to divide schizophrenia followed the route of identifying subgroups of patients and is as old as the disorder itself. When Kraepelin created the concept of schizophrenia in 1896 he constructed it out of three existing disorders: catatonia, described twenty years earlier by Kahlbaum (1874); hebephrenia, described by Kahlbaum's protegé, Heckers (1871, see Sedler, 1985); and dementia paranoides, described by another of Kahlbaum's followers, Kraepelin himself. Although outwardly very different, Kraepelin argued that the three disorders were all variants of a single disease entity, first because they all followed a similar course ending in 'a more or less well marked mental enfeeblement', and secondly because 'between them there are such numerous transitions that in spite of all efforts it appears impossible at present to delimit them sharply'. To the three original subtypes Bleuler (1911) then added a fourth, simple schizophrenia, a state of progressive deterioration without any florid symptoms which had originally been described by Diem (1903).

The paranoid, hebephrenic, catatonic and simple forms of schizophrenia did not in any way segregate patients according to the presence or absence of thought disorder. Although incoherence of speech was regarded as one of the characteristic symptoms of hebephrenic schizophrenia, Kraepelin considered that it was also common in paranoid schizophrenia along with the defining symptoms of this subtype, delusions and hallucinations. Thought disorder could also be seen in catatonic schizophrenia, where it sometimes took a very severe form. Even some of the patients in Diem's original series of simple schizophrenic patients were described as being diffuse, vague, circumstantial and too detailed in their speech (Pomarol-Clotet, unpublished M.Phil. thesis).

By 1913 Kraepelin had modified the original four-way subclassification of schizophrenia. As well as dividing paranoid schizophrenia into mild and severe forms ('paranoid dementia mitis' and 'paranoid dementia gravis') and adding a number of groups where there was marked depression and elation, he felt it necessary to add 'a last very peculiar group of cases . . . characterized by an unusually striking disorder of expression in speech with relatively little impairment of the remaining psychic activities'. His description of this form of schizophrenia, which he called confusional speech dementia, is reproduced in Box 2.1.

Box 2.1 Kraepelin's speech confused subtype of schizophrenia

(From Kraepelin, 1913a)

Commencement. Sometimes a gradual failing with restlessness and silly actions, sometimes a moody condition with irritating hallucinations, ideas of persecution and serious attempts at suicide forms the beginning. Often the malady is developed in short attacks, between which there are remissions of considerable extent and lasting for years. Some patients sink to vagrants; one became a crier at market-stalls. But by degrees, now and then apparently within a fairly short time, the extremely remarkable morbid symptom is developed, which characterizes these patients above everything, confusion of speech.

General Features. Perception and memory usually show no considerable disorder, as far as can be judged from the utterances of the patients; in any case the patients are clear about their place of abode, also about time relations, recognize quite correctly the people in their surroundings, even though they often give them wonderful names to which they usually adhere. Auditory hallucinations appear still to persist, but play no recognizable part in the psychic life of the patients and are not further worked up. Indications also of delusions appear, ideas of persecution, complaints about influences at night, 'interpolations', and along with these there are exalted ideas. All these delusions are, however, extraordinarily vague, are only produced occasionally in often changing, often half-jocular, form, and acquire no influence over the rest of thought and activity. The patients are mentally active, accessible, show interest in their surroundings, often also follow the events of the day quite well.

Conduct and outward behaviour are reasonable, sometimes a little affected, submissive, or whimsical; the patients have the tendency to adopt all sorts of little peculiarities from which they are only with difficulty dissuaded. At the same time they are as a rule very useful, diligent and clever workers, who occupy themselves without assistance, but like to go their own way, ward off every interference in their doings, will not work with others, for the most part fulfil their obligations with great carefulness, but probably also once in a while do something quite nonsensical.

Speech. As soon as they are addressed, they frequently answer with great vivacity and immediately take up the attitude of a lecturer. To simple questions put with emphasis they generally give a short and suitable answer. Or perhaps that throng of disconnected utterances, which was described before, begins immediately, at most after the first still tolerably intelligible sentences. It is produced in flowing speech and with a certain satisfaction on the part of the patient. These utterances are mostly quite *unintelligible* and are richly interspersed with speech *derailments* and *neologisms*. Often the current can only be brought to a standstill by the interference of the questioner and can again be immediately put in motion by renewed questioning. Sometimes it is possible from the behaviour of the patient and from detached, less nonsensical parts of the talk, to make at least very vague guesses what thoughts he wishes perhaps to express, stories of long ago, complaints, boasting, taunts, but all hidden in the most bewildering phrases which abruptly digress into the most remote domains of thought.

An example of such utterances is given in the following letter:

The sentimental vocation of the Welschneureuther citizens requires above everything that after the sublime birthday festival of his Majesty the illustrious King William Charles, all his spiritual powers should be collected in order to do justice to their pastoral intercession in the Lord. So forty respected stormpatriots in view of the repeal of the statutes of the University of Erlangen have to-day taken it upon them to confirm as first retrospective negative in analogical-patriotic sense. To place at the most gracious disposition of his Majesty the Art. I of the Welschneureuther constitution, consisting in combustible available war-material, further most obediently to stop the most notorious dealings as intercourse with cattle, sheep and turkeys. Now in order that the sublime royal company cannot be subjected to any competition from the neighbouring states in transportable tempers all to be recommended to indulgence, we swear by the profit of enhanced merchandise only to serve each alone, only then to break off a consequence of the balance of the nineteenth century to be drawn periodically and mechanically, when we shall be able to be expectantly deceived in our opinions towards our august ruler and regarded as a useful adviser of a healthy antiquarian museum and so on.

The severity, with which the phenomenon of confusion of speech appears, is subjected to great fluctuation. Many patients are usually able to express themselves at first quite intelligibly, but fall into their nonsensical talk as soon as one speaks for a longer time with them or when they become excited. Further, periods are frequently noticed which recur with approximate periodicity, in which the patients are more ill-tempered or excited, and then become much more easily confused in speech; it is exactly this peculiarity which completely corresponds with the observations in the other terminal states of dementia praecox. But lastly a state of confusion of speech may again disappear even after existing for many years, till only slight traces remain noticeable during excitement. That, for

Box 2.1 (cont.)

example, was the case of the patient from whom the letter given above originated; he applied later in a quite correct way for a post. At the same time there is here certainly no question of real recovery. Lack of insight into their morbid state and lack of judgment, restlessness and aimlessness in work, a tendency to use high-sounding phrases and superficiality of the emotions remain behind even in favourable cases.

A speech confused subtype of schizophrenia also featured in the even more complicated subtyping developed by Kraepelin's contemporary and rival, Wernicke. According to him, it was only in the early stages that the clinical presentations of schizophrenia were amorphous and overlapping, and as the disease progressed these gradually crystallised into over thirty stable presentations, in each of which one or a small number of symptoms predominated to the exclusion of most others. This alternative tradition was kept alive by Wernicke's followers Kleist (Fish 1957), and later Leonard (1979), and still has its adherents today (e.g. Astrup, 1979). The speech-confused subtype has been preserved in all these classifications as schizophasia, although it has sometimes been divided into two forms, and it remains considerably better known than such alleged entities as affect-laden paraphrenia, insipid hebephrenia and proskinetic catatonia.

Kraepelin's expanded classification failed to stand the test of time, and the Wernicke–Kleist–Leonhard system never had any more than a handful of supporters. Even the original four-way subdivision has not stood up particularly well to experimental scrutiny. For example, Carpenter *et al.* (1976) applied the statistical technique of cluster analysis to a sample of 600 acute schizophrenic patients, whose symptoms were rated using an early version of the Present State Examination (see Chapter 1). Cluster analysis partitions the members of a presumptively heterogeneous population into more homogeneous subgroups, according to the similarities individual subjects show to each other and/or their dissimilarities from other subjects. They found that four clusters accounted for almost all the patients. The first two were highly reminiscent of paranoid and hebephrenic schizophrenia: the former was characterised by persecutory delusions, auditory hallucinations, flattened affect and the latter by these symptoms plus social withdrawal, thought disorder, inappropriate affect, disturbed behaviour and self-neglect. However, the remaining two clusters showed little resemblance to catatonic and simple schizophrenia. Patients in one type had high ratings on delusions, hallucinations and neurotic symptoms, and tended to have good insight. In the other type the predominant psychotic symptom was visual hallucinations.

Today everyone accepts that the clinical presentations of schizophrenia are infinitely variable and any alleged subtypes are ideals which shade into one another via innumerable transitions, just as Kraepelin described. In fact, it is almost axiomatic that any schizophrenic symptom can be seen in any form of schizophrenia, or at least in any form apart from simple schizophrenia. While patients with classical paranoid, classical hebephrenic and (rarely) classical catatonic schizophrenia are sometimes encountered, somewhere along the way the concept of a speech confused subtype of schizophrenia has been consigned to oblivion.

Subdividing schizophrenia II: positive and negative symptoms

The precise moment when the focus of attempts to subdivide schizophrenia shifted from groups of patients to groups of symptoms is easy to pinpoint. In 1980 Crow published a theoretical article entitled 'Molecular pathology of schizophrenia: more than one disease process?'. In this, partly based on his own group's findings, he proposed that the pathological process which gave rise to the florid symptoms of acute schizophrenia was different from that underlying the features of chronic illness. The psychosis-inducing effects of drugs like amphetamine coupled with the therapeutic effectiveness of neuroleptic drugs linked acute schizophrenia to a neurochemical disturbance, specifically an excess of dopamine (Johnstone et al., 1978). In contrast, chronic schizophrenic patients were relatively resistant to the effects of amphetamine, and some of them showed cognitive impairment similar to that seen in organic brain disease (Crow and Mitchell, 1975). The first CT scan study of schizophrenia, which Johnstone et al. (1976) had recently carried out, also provided evidence of a brain abnormality in chronic patients, lateral ventricular enlargement. He then went on to articulate his groundbreaking distinction:

It seems that two syndromes can be distinguished in those diseases currently described as schizophrenic and that each may be associated with a specific pathological process. The first (the type I syndrome, equivalent to 'acute schizophrenia' and characterised by the positive symptoms – delusions, hallucinations, and thought disorder) is in some way associated with a change in dopaminergic transmission; the second process (the type II syndrome, equivalent to the 'defect state' and characterised by negative symptoms – affective flattening and poverty of speech) is unrelated to dopaminergic transmission, but may be associated with intellectual impairment and, perhaps, structural changes in the brain. Type I symptoms are reversible; type II symptoms, which are more difficult to define, may indicate a component of irreversibility. The former predict a potential response to neuroleptics; the latter are more closely associated with a poor long-term outcome. Episodes of type I symptoms may be followed by development of the type II syndrome, and both may be present together. Type II symptoms, however, define a group of illnesses of graver prognosis.

What Crow meant by molecular may not have been entirely clear, and his type I and type II terminology was destined to be short lived, but a novel and potentially important way of identifying subdivisions in schizophrenia had arrived.

The matter-of-fact way in which Crow used the terms positive and negative symptoms implied that this was not the first time they had been employed. In fact, according to Berrios (1985, 1991), the history of the positive/negative distinction stretches back to the last century when Reynolds, a physician, employed positive and negative to divide neurological phenomena into those consisting of 'the excess or alteration of vital properties' and those understandable as the 'the negation of vital properties'. Several claims have been staked for the first modern usage of the terms in schizophrenia. However, the honour probably belongs to Wing and Brown (1970), who in the course of a study on the effects of institutionalisation incidentally observed that the symptoms of chronic schizophrenia appeared to fall into two independent clusters. One of these was florid or positive symptoms, which included delusions, hallucinations, thought disorder, overactivity and various forms of odd behaviour. The other, which they called the clinical poverty syndrome, consisted of social withdrawal, affective flattening, lack of volition, poverty of speech and slowness and underactivity.

On the heels of Wing and Brown (1970), and on the basis of a completely different line of reasoning, Strauss *et al.* (1974) made the crucial phenomenological distinction that positive symptoms were distinguished by the presence of an abnormal phenomenon and negative symptoms were distinguished by the absence or diminution of a normal function. The key section of their paper, which also hinted at some of the problems the concept was subsequently to face, is reproduced in Box 2.2.

Andreasen, (1982) added the finishing touches, giving a detailed specification of the two classes of symptom.[1] This was easy for positive symptoms: everyone agreed these comprised delusions, hallucinations, some kinds of thought disorder and, insofar as anyone thought about them, catatonic symptoms. It was less easy for negative symptoms. The triad of lack of volition, poverty of speech and flattening of affect identified by Crow and other authors seemed somehow formulaic, almost a shorthand for what was almost certainly a richer vein of

---

[1] As all the original authors recognised, but which has sometimes been misunderstood since, positive and negative symptoms are groups of symptoms that run together and not groups of patients. While some schizophrenic patients have only positive or only negative symptoms, the majority show a combination of both, either simultaneously or at different times.

Box 2.2 The first modern definition of positive and negative symptoms

(From Strauss *et al.*, 1974)

These data suggest the utility of postulating that three major types of processes underlie schizophrenic symptoms and signs. These three hypothetical processes can be arrived at by grouping the six kinds of symptoms into three categories: positive symptoms, negative symptoms, and disorders in relating. The terms positive and negative symptoms were first used by Hughlings Jackson (1887) in his evolution-dissolution theory of nervous function to describe manifestations of postulated underlying mechanisms. We use these terms here primarily descriptively without necessarily implying Jackson's theoretical conceptions, but find the terms useful because symptoms within each of the groups appear to have some important basic similarities in their relationship to antecedents and outcome. In this way, the concepts of positive and negative symptoms may help shed light on the basic pathological processes involved in schizophrenia.

As Jackson described them, positive symptoms are those that have the appearance of being active processes – for example, delusions, hallucinations, and catatonic motor phenomena. In a discussion of this group of symptoms, Snezhnevsky considers them similar also because of their relative flexibility. Negative symptoms, on the other hand, involve primarily absence of normal functions. In schizophrenia, negative symptoms include such phenomena as blunting of affect, apathy, and certain kinds of formal thought disorder, such as blocking. Snezhnevsky describes the inflexibility of this group of symptoms.

There is some question about the consistency of these concepts, especially about how to categorize those manifestations of schizophrenia that reflect absence of normal function but are also flexible such as a transitory episode of loosening of associations. Nevertheless, the basic concepts appear valuable enough to justify attempts to apply them further. In this report, the criterion of flexibility will be given priority where necessary over the criterion of absence of a normal function, which in any case is the more difficult characteristic to establish. Positive symptoms will be considered as including from the six symptom areas disorders of content of thought and perception, certain types of form of thought (e.g., distractibility) and certain behaviors (e.g., catatonic motor disorders). Negative symptoms will be considered as including from the six symptom areas blunting of affect, apathy, and certain kinds of formal thought disorder, such as blocking. Disorders of relating will be considered separately. Of the six types of symptoms and signs, one, lack of insight, is obviously important but does not fit neatly into any category; nor are there many data available regarding its antecedents or prognostic implications.

abnormality. Drawing on her own clinical experience, plus an earlier rating scale she had devised for affective flattening (Andreasen et al., 1979b), she developed a scale, the Scale for the Assessment of Negative Symptoms (SANS) (Andreasen, 1982). This identified five categories of negative symptoms: alogia, affective flattening, avolition-apathy, anhedonia-asociality and attentional impairment. Of particular relevance to this chapter was her category of alogia, which included poverty of speech, poverty of content of speech, blocking and increased latency of responding.

Andreasen and Olsen (1982) carried out one of the first studies directed to establishing that schizophrenic symptoms did actually segregate into two syndromes. They did this by rating a wide range of symptoms in a group of fifty-two acute schizophrenic patients and analysing the pattern of intercorrelations. They rated negative symptoms using the SANS and positive symptoms by means of an early version of the corresponding Schedule for Assessment of Positive Symptoms (SAPS). This included items for different types of delusions and hallucinations, a shortened form of the TLC scale, plus measures of bizarre behaviour and catatonic symptoms. The correlations between global ratings on each of the five classes of negative symptoms were all found to be significant, with the exception of that between affective flattening and attentional impairment.

Among positive symptoms, delusions and hallucinations were significantly correlated with each other, but the correlations between both of these and thought disorder scores, while in the expected direction, were not significant. Bizarre behaviour and catatonic motor behaviour were not correlated with either positive or negative symptoms in any consistent way. As predicted, all types of negative symptoms were either uncorrelated with or significantly inversely correlated with all types of positive symptoms.

These findings were typical of a number of subsequent studies with sample sizes ranging from thirty-two to over 500 (see McKenna, 1994). One symptom, however, did not fit neatly into the positive:negative framework. This was inappropriate affect, which Andreasen included in her earlier reliability and validity study of her rating scale for affective flattening (Andreasen, 1979b) and her final full scale for negative symptoms (Andreasen, 1982). This was despite the fact that she found it correlated poorly with other measures of affective flattening, such as unchanging facial expression, poor eye contact and emotional unresponsivity, prompting her to comment that 'it may be a weak measure of negative symptoms'. Together with the weak association between thought disorder and other positive symptoms, this minor irregularity was to assume major significance when a more sophisticated way of exploring the correlations among schizophrenic symptoms – factor analysis – began to be employed.

Liddle's three syndromes

Factor analysis takes the pattern of intercorrelations among a set of variables, in this case schizophrenic symptoms, and aims to reduce them to a smaller set of underlying variables, or factors, which account for most of the variation in the original data (see Box 2.3). In the first study of this type in schizophrenia,[2] Liddle (1987a) applied factor analysis to the symptoms shown by a group of forty stable chronic patients. He rated their symptoms using Andreasen's SANS and SAPS scales, or the Comprehensive Assessment of Symptoms and History (CASH) (Andreasen, 1987) as they were collectively referred to. The analysis was carried out on individual symptoms rather than on global scores for delusions, hallucinations, alogia, etc., in order to avoid having to make assumptions about what should be regarded as positive or negative – inappropriate affect being a case in point. In addition, he only included those items in the SANS which were unequivocally symptoms, for example poverty of speech, blocking and unchanging facial expression, and not those which might be regarded as measures of performance in daily life, such as poor self-care and impersistence in work or school and relationships with friends and peers. For statistical reasons, Liddle also excluded symptoms which were present in less than 10% of the patients.

Box 2.3 What is factor analysis?

(From Blashfield, 1984)

Factor analysis attempts to account for the pattern of correlations among scores on a set of variables (for example symptoms) in terms of one or more non-observable variables, or factors. Its history is inextricably bound up with the history of intelligence testing. Spearman noted that scores on all of a range of tests of ability were positively correlated with one another – in other words if a person performed well on one test he or she was likely to perform well on another – and developed a technique whereby a general factor g could be isolated from the matrix of correlations between the individual tests. Spearman's g was to all intents and purposes IQ.

One way of conceptualising factor analysis is as a procedure for re-organising a matrix of correlations to find groups of variables that vary together – i.e. the intercorrelations within a particular group are high, whereas the correlations with variables outside the group are low. This is achieved mathematically, and there are

---

[2] As customary with scientific advances, Liddle's study was not the first factor analysis of schizophrenic symptoms. Both Andreasen (Andreasen and Olsen, 1982; Andreasen and Grove, 1986a) and Bilder *et al.* (1985) had carried out similar analyses, with less clear-cut findings in the former and without recognising its significance in the latter.

Box 2.3 (cont.)

many different techniques for doing so. In one of the most widely used methods, a linear combination of the observed variables is first formed which accounts for as much of the variation as possible in the original data. After this first factor is created, the variance associated with it is removed from the correlation matrix. This generally reduces the values of the correlations among the variables. Then a second factor is created, the variance associated with it removed, and so on. The correlations between the observed variables and a particular factor are referred to as their loadings on the factor.

The process of estimating factors and forming a revised correlation matrix can be repeated many times; factor analysis will generate as many factors as there are variables in the correlation matrix. However, the aim is to select a small number of factors which account for a large amount of the variation in the original data. There are a number of rules for optimising the number of factors chosen. One of the most widely used is simply to choose all factors which have so-called eigenvalues of greater than 1 (the eigenvalue is a measure of the amount of variance in the total sample accounted for by each factor). Another is the scree test, which requires plotting the eigenvalues for each of the factors and drawing a straight line along the smallest as shown; the first value that is markedly above this line dictates the cutoff point.

Whether the loading of an individual variable on a particular factor is considered significant is dictated by convention. One of the most widely used conventions is a value of 0.5 or greater, but there are no hard and fast rules.

The above procedure isolates factors which account for progressively less of the variance in the data. As an alternative, the factors obtained can be manipulated or 'rotated' to minimise the number of variables with high loadings on any one given

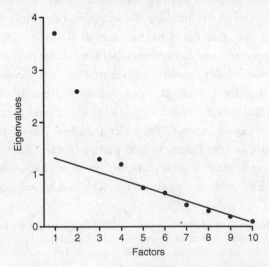

factor. This has the effect of finding factors that best capture different variables with high (and low) loadings, and so makes it as easy as possible to identify each variable with a single factor. The most frequently used rotations are orthogonal (in which the new factors keep being completely uncorrelated). However, allowing some degree of between factors (non-orthogonal or oblique rotation) may help in better grouping the observed variables.

The factor analysis produced three rather than two factors. These were weakly correlated with each other, suggesting that they were independent rather than associated or mutually exclusive. The three factors are shown in Table 2.1. Two were immediately recognisable as positive and negative symptoms. The former (which Liddle termed reality distortion) had high loadings on auditory hallucinations, delusions of persecution and delusions of reference. The latter (which Liddle termed psychomotor poverty) loaded heavily on poverty of speech,

Table 2.1 Three syndromes obtained by factor analysis of CASH ratings in forty chronic schizophrenic patients,

(From Liddle, 1987a reproduced with permission)

Symptoms	Factor 1	Factor 2	Factor 3
Psychomotor poverty syndrome			
Poverty of speech	0.80	−0.01	−0.03
Decreased spontaneous movement	0.95	−0.04	−0.03
Unchanging facial expression	0.85	−0.01	0.05
Paucity of expressive gesture	0.97	0.02	−0.04
Affective non-responsivity	0.82	0.02	0.00
Lack of vocal inflection	0.90	−0.20	−0.05
Disorganisation syndrome			
Inappropriate affect	0.19	0.84	0.09
Poverty of content of speech	−0.08	0.57	0.01
Tangentiality	−0.05	0.94	0.03
Derailment	−0.05	0.94	0.04
Pressure of speech	−0.10	0.61	0.08
Distractibility	0.00	0.81	0.01
Reality distortion syndrome			
Voices speak to patient	0.04	−0.07	0.67
Delusions of persecution	−0.19	0.06	0.51
Delusions of reference	0.13	0.04	0.84
Somatic delusions	−0.03	−0.03	0.03

decreased spontaneous movement, unchanging facial expression, paucity of expressive gestures, affective non-responsivity and lack of vocal inflection. The third factor was composed of thought disorder items, tangentiality, derailment, pressure of speech and distractibility, plus poverty of content of speech and also inappropriate affect. Liddle termed this factor disorganisation, a term which, unlike reality distortion and psychomotor poverty, has been universally adopted.

Liddle obtained similar results when he used ratings from the Present State Examination instead of the CASH, and when the exercise was repeated on a different sample of patients (Liddle and Barnes, 1990). Numerous further studies, large and small, carried out on acute and chronic schizophrenic patients, and using factor analysis with and without rotation, have confirmed the finding (see Thompson and Meltzer, 1993; Andreasen et al., 1995; plus Phillips et al., 1991; Shtasel et al., 1992; Malla et al., 1993; Sarai and Matsunaga, 1993; Gureje et al., 1995; Johnstone and Frith, 1996; Vásquez-Barquero et al., 1996; Arora et al., 1997). Confirmatory factor analyses, which mathematically test the goodness-of-fit of different models, have invariably reached the conclusion that more than two factors are needed to satisfactorily account for the correlations among schizophrenic symptoms, and have found little to choose between three- and four-factor models (Brekke et al., 1994; Peralta et al., 1994; Dollfus and Everitt, 1998; Smith et al., 1998).

Stuart et al. (1999) raised a late objection to the three syndrome model, pointing out that many of the above studies deviated from Liddle's original methodology by using scores for entire categories of symptoms rather than scores for the individual symptoms themselves. Typically, what these studies entered into the factor analysis were CASH global ratings for delusions, hallucinations, thought disorder, bizarre behaviour and the five main subdivisions of negative symptoms. This necessarily constrained the number of factors that could be produced, or as Stuart et al. put it, 'it is perhaps not surprising that only two factors are required to explain the correlations between the four positive symptoms, with a third to account for the correlations between negative symptom ratings'.

Dealing with this objection runs up against the problem that factor analysis should ideally use a ratio of subjects (i.e. patients) to variables (i.e. symptoms) of 4:1 to 5:1. Table 2.2 summarises the small number of factor analytic studies that have used individual schizophrenic symptoms, and which have not violated this rule by too great a margin, either by employing large sample sizes or by utilising the kinds of measures to reduce the number of individual symptoms employed by Liddle (1987a) in his original study. All the studies isolated factors recognisable as positive, negative and disorganisation syndromes. Two found four rather than three factors (Shtasel et al., 1992; Arora et al., 1997), but in both cases the extra factor simply split the positive or negative symptom factor. One other study found

Table 2.2 Factor analytic studies of schizophrenia using individual symptoms

Study	Sample size	Symptom ratings	No. of factors	Variance accounted for (%)	Positive symptoms	Negative symptoms	Disorgan- isation	Comment
Shtasel et al. (1992)	107	SAPS/SANS/ BPRS	4	33	✓ [see comment]	✓	✓	Delusions and hallucinations loaded on two factors.
Malla et al. (1993)	155	SAPS/SANS	3	46	✓	✓	✓	–
Thompson and Meltzer (1995)	131	SADS/PSE	3	76	✓	✓	✓	'Other delusions' loaded on disorganisation factor.
Cardno et al. (1996)	102	OPCRIT	3/5	35	✓	✓	✓ [see comment]	Catatonia loaded on negative factor. Using scree test instead of eigenvalue > 1 divided positive syndrome into three factors after rotation.
Arora et al. (1997)	80	SAPS/SANS	4	47	✓	✓ [see comment]	✓	Used eigenvalue of 2. Negative symptoms in two factors.

Notes: SAPS/SANS – Scales for the Assessment of Positive and Negative symptoms, BPRS – Brief Psychiatric Rating Scale, PANSS – Positive and Negative Syndrome Scale, SADS – Schedule for Affective Disorders and Schizophrenia. PSE – Present State Examination, OPCRIT – Operational Checklist for Psychotic Illness.

five factors (Cardno *et al.*, 1996). However, this was only found using a more liberal cutoff for the inclusion of factors (the scree test); use of a more conservative criterion (eigenvalues above 1) resulted in the standard positive, negative and disorganisation factors.

The three syndrome model of schizophrenia is difficult to resist in the face of this united front of findings. While it is true, as Kendell (1975) has pointed out, that there is no necessity for the number of factors produced in a factor analysis to correspond to the number of underlying sources of variation, the consistency with which the technique has segregated groups of positive, negative and disorganisation symptoms in schizophrenia makes a strong case that they reflect true natural cleavages in the disorder. If this is accepted, then there is no escaping the further conclusion that thought disorder is a discrete syndrome in schizophrenia, with everything this entails – from its different elements being intrinsically associated with each other, to the possibility that a single pathology underlies all its manifestations. Why this pathological process should give rise not just to thought disorder but also symptoms like inappropriate affect and bizarre behaviour remains mysterious, but it is not unprecedented – the co-occurrence of thought disorder, inappropriate affect and bizarre behaviour had registered on psychiatry as hebephrenia even before schizophrenia was identified as a disorder.

Positive and negative thought disorder?

A year before Crow (1980) brought positive and negative symptoms centre stage, Andreasen (1979c) had proposed that it might be useful 'to conceptualize "thought disorder" as consisting of two basic types "positive" or "negative"'. According to this line of reasoning, positive thought disorder was characterised by pressure of speech, tangentiality, derailment, incoherence and illogicality, and represented an overabundance of thoughts, as typically seen in acute schizophrenic patients. Negative thought disorder or alogia, on the other hand, was characterised by poverty of speech and poverty of content of speech and conveyed the sense of intellectual emptiness and apathy seen in many chronic schizophrenic patients.

The pattern of intercorrelations among the items of the TLC scale that Andreasen (1979a,c) found in the study described in the last chapter in some ways tended to support this distinction. Among 113 psychotic patients ratings of derailment, tangentiality, loss of goal, pressure of speech, illogicality and incoherence were all significantly correlated with each other. In contrast, poverty of speech showed no correlations with these or any other items in the scale.

However, the picture was less clear-cut with respect to the other main alleged element of negative thought disorder, poverty of content of speech. This was not significantly correlated with poverty of speech, but showed significant correlations with several of the intercorrelated group of positive thought disorder items. Clanging and distractible speech showed few significant correlations with any of the items in the scale, positive or negative.

Not too much can be concluded from these results, since the sample was made up of a mixture of schizophrenic, manic and depressed patients. Subsequently, though, Harvey et al. (1992) carried out essentially the same study on a sample of 142 newly admitted male inpatients with a diagnosis of schizophrenia. Two independent assessors made thought disorder ratings using the TLC scale, and consensus ratings were derived from these. For a complicated set of reasons, Harvey et al. chose to include only scores on eight of the TLC scale items in their correlational analysis, but fortunately these were the important ones. Their findings are shown in Table 2.3. It can be seen that, as in Andreasen's (1979a,c) study, tangentiality, derailment and incoherence formed a tightly intercorrelated group of abnormalities, with the first two of these also being highly correlated with loss of goal. Poverty of speech, on the other hand, showed inverse correlations with all the TLC items apart from poverty of content of speech, where there was a small but significant positive correlation of 0.22. Poverty of content of speech also showed significant correlations with tangentiality and derailment, and to a slightly lower degree with incoherence, circumstantiality and loss of goal.

These studies confirmed the widely accepted view that poverty of speech was not part of the syndrome of thought disorder characterised by abnormalities such as derailment, tangentiality, loss of goal, illogicality and incoherence. Poverty of content of speech, however, appeared to occupy a more ambiguous position, aligning itself both with 'positive' thought disorder items and with the main constituent of 'negative' thought disorder, poverty of speech. This statistical ambiguity mirrors Wing's phenomenological ambivalence about poverty of content of speech. As described in Chapter 1, he (Wing, 1961) originally considered this to be a variant of poverty of speech, but by the time the definitive 9th Edition (Wing et al., 1974) was published it had become one of a trio of overlapping abnormalities which also included incoherence and flight of ideas.

Wing's later formulation, which essentially made poverty of content of speech the mild end of a continuum of positive thought disorder, has a certain amount of intuitive appeal. This is because, in practice, deciding whether a stretch of schizophrenic speech shows poverty of content rather than derailment and loss of goal depends on quite subjective judgements about the presence or absence of topic shift, whether the goal is reached and so on. At the other end of the spectrum it can sometimes be difficult to decide whether the abnormality is occurring

Table 2.3 Intercorrelations of thought disorder items in 142 schizophrenic patients

(Reprinted from Harvey et al., 1992, with permission from Elsevier, copyright 1992)

	Poverty of speech	Poverty of content	Pressure of speech	Tangentiality	Derailment	Incoherence	Circumstantiality
Poverty of speech	–						
Poverty of content	0.22**	–					
Pressure of speech	-0.32***	0.10	–				
Tangentiality	-0.20*	0.45***	0.32***	–			
Derailment	-0.22**	0.44***	0.32***	0.71***	–		
Incoherence	-0.10	0.35***	0.09	0.51***	0.59***	–	
Circumstantiality	-0.09	0.34***	0.05	0.20*	0.31***	0.27**	–
Loss of goal	-0.15	0.35***	0.23**	0.54***	0.45***	0.19*	0.27**

Note: * P < 0.05; ** P < 0.01; *** P < 0.001.

predominantly from sentence to sentence, as in derailment, loss of goal, etc., or whether individual sentences themselves fail to make sense, justifying a designation of incoherence. This apparent continuity can be illustrated by the three extracts shown in Box 2.4. Taken individually, these appear to be respectable examples of poverty of content of speech, derailment and incoherence; however, they are all from the same patient.

Box 2.4 The apparent continuity between different degrees of thought disorder

(From Laws *et al.*, 1999 and unpublished data from Oh *et al.*, 2002)

Poverty of content of speech
Patient describing how he feels:
I feel quite well, but I keep expecting to get well, to be made well, but I never seem to get well and, you know, every day I put in, I expect the following day to get better and to be well and doing things and achieving goals and aims and all that sort of thing, but I just sort of get the pills every day and I don't seem to make much progress. But I would like to be, you know, feel well in myself and I would like to be talking more to people and socialising and all that kind of thing but, um, maybe it's because I haven't seen an awful lot of the doctors over the period, I don't know. I feel that talking to a doctor helps, you know, with your problems and everything. Um, the way things are going I am hopeful for things to come. I have achieved all I have wanted to, but there is a lot more, you know, and I have got the next six months to go and I have got to do more than I have done in the last six months. I want to do a lot, but it is just getting well, you know. It's relying on doctors and nurses for help and sort of... I wouldn't be promolgurating your illness or anything else... that's partly my intention.
What does promolgurate mean?
Well it's conjuring up your own beliefs and ideas and theories and ideas and that and putting them in practice in making the world go round, sort of thing.

Tangentiality, derailment, loss of goal, clanging
How are you?
To relate to people about new-found... talk about statistical ideology. Er, I find that it's like starting in respect of ideology, ideals change and ideals present ideology and... new entertainments... new, new attainments. And the more one talks about like, ideal totalitananism or hotelatarianism, it's like you want new ideas to be formulated, so that everyone can benefit in mankind, so we can all

Box 2.4 (cont.)

live in our ideal heaven. Presumably that's what we still want, and with these ideas it can be brought about. I find the . . . it's like a rose garden.

Incoherence

Patient explaining why he responded 'true' in response to *Forks are used for fuel*, in a semantic verification task:

Yes, they add up and kind of like a solution. It's say, it's an equine or equinox, like fungi. Something in the brain tells you it's a high number. Bacteriology, a numerate number, it's a particle, therefore it contains solution is to answer the right question. A fork is a solution, an aqueous solution. Fork in a kettle, something bottle, do hairs bristle on a comb or fungi? It could be naval or positive solution ratified like a kettle, if kettle is the right answer. It could be 5th or 7th one, right? Brown aqueous solution inside the kettle.

After Andreasen and her co-workers (Miller *et al.*, 1993) found, as Liddle (1987a) had previously, that poverty of speech was associated with negative symptoms and poverty of content with disorganisation in a factor analytic study, they conceded that negative thought disorder might be composed of two separate and somewhat independent factors. Almost immediately, however, they (Andreasen *et al.*, 1995) about turned, arguing that poverty of speech and poverty of content of speech were conceptually linked by their fundamental characteristic of intellectual emptiness, but for purely practical reasons could not be rated together – the former specified a reduction in speech and the latter required speech to be adequate in quantity. At the present time, this is where the matter rests, with what may or may not be a fudge.

The factor structure of thought disorder

It seems inherently unlikely that all of the elements of thought disorder included by Andreasen (1979a) – which merely have in common the fact that they can be reliably identified – are the final word on the make-up of the syndrome. Such being the case, if the application of factor analysis can reveal an unsuspected deep structure in the symptoms of schizophrenia, perhaps it can do the same for the symptoms of thought disorder. Along the way, it might also be able to shed some further light on how poverty of content of speech fits into the picture. So far, factor analysis of TLC scale ratings has only been carried out twice, but in studies whose results have shown intriguing similarities.

Andreasen and Grove (1986b) factor analysed TLC scale ratings on one hundred patients. Unfortunately, the sample was not ideal for the present purposes, being

Table 2.4 Factor analysis of thought disorder ratings in 100 (schizophrenic, schizoaffective and manic) patients

(From Andreasen and Grove, 1986)

Variable	Fluent disorganisation	Emptiness	Linguistic control
Poverty of content	0.24	0.61	0.05
Poverty of speech	−0.59	0.42	0.17
Pressure of speech	0.65	−0.46	−0.08
Derailment	0.77	0.025	−0.11
Incoherence	0.63	0.36	−0.09
Illogicality	0.55	0.13	0.26
Word approximations	0.50	0.26	0.36
Circumstantiality	0.50	−0.49	−0.02
Loss of goal	0.74	0.02	−0.24
Perseveration	0.75	−0.05	0.14
Clanging	0.44	0.32	−0.47
Distractible speech	0.43	−0.16	−0.21
Stilted speech	0.53	0.09	0.53
Self reference	0.27	−0.15	0.67
Tangentiality	0.25	0.46	−0.13
Neologisms	0.23	0.24	−0.35
Echolalia	0.10	−0.28	−0.22
Blocking	0.04	0.10	0.29
% of variance	25.5	9.7	8.9

made up of fifty patients with schizophrenia, twenty-five with schizoaffective disorder and twenty-five with mania. As shown in Table 2.4, three factors were identified. The first factor had high loadings on pressure of speech, derailment, incoherence, illogicality, word approximations, circumstantiality, loss of goal, perseveration and stilted speech. Clanging and distractible speech loaded on this factor at 0.43 and 0.44, slightly below the widely used though arbitrary cutoff of 0.5. Poverty of speech had a negative loading of −0.59. This factor thus captured many of the items conventionally associated with thought disorder. Andreasen and Grove termed it 'fluent disorganisation'.

The second factor loaded at greater than 0.5 only on poverty of content of speech. Poverty of speech had a marginally subthreshold loading at 0.42. Tangentiality also showed a just subthreshold loading of 0.46. Despite the loading on this last abnormality, Andreasen and Grove called this factor 'emptiness'.

Factor 3 loaded on stilted speech and self reference. Andreasen and Grove noted that the components of this factor occurred so infrequently that the factor could not be considered an important one.

Peralta *et al.* (1992) carried out a similar study on a sample of 115 acute admissions with a diagnosis of schizophrenia. Factor analysis yielded seven factors with eigenvalues greater than 1, of which they considered the first five to be valid, based on an analysis of their internal consistency. Factor 1 was similar to Andreasen and Grove's first factor, loading on derailment, loss of goal, tangentiality, illogical thinking and circumstantiality; incoherence also had a loading of 0.42. Factor 2 loaded on poverty of speech, poverty of content of speech and perseveration. The third factor loaded on stilted speech and word approximations, the fourth factor on neologisms and clanging, and the fifth factor on blocking and distractible speech.

These two studies both extracted a large factor, which included most of the abnormalities customarily regarded as the main constituents of thought disorder and went beyond the group of tightly intercorrelated positive thought disorder items indentified by Andreasen (1979a, c) and Harvey *et al.* (1992) in their correlational studies. The remaining TLC items were distributed among a number of other factors, either separately or in small, not very meaningful groupings. In both analyses poverty of content of speech segregated with poverty of speech in one of these ancillary groupings – definitely in one study and equivocally in the other – in what looks suspiciously like a negative thought disorder factor.

Conclusion

This chapter has tried to address the validity of thought disorder by asking the question of whether its different elements 'are intrinsically more closely related to each other than to other symptoms', to borrow a phrase Bleuler (1911) used in connection with catatonic symptoms. It is somewhat surprising that this question can be answered at all, and more surprising that the construct acquits itself so well. Factor analysis of the symptoms of schizophrenia isolates a disorganisation syndrome, of which thought disorder is the major constituent. Factor analysis of the symptoms of thought disorder reveals that, on the whole, its individual elements do run together in the way expected of a syndrome, although, as expected, this syndrome does not include poverty of speech.

Beyond this, factor analysis may or may not have revealed divisions within thought disorder, but it has certainly exposed a division among those who study it. There are those who believe that poverty of content of speech is a form of positive, fluent, disorganised speech, which probably represents the mild end of a continuum at the other end of which is incoherence. And then there are those who believe that it is a negative symptom closely related to poverty of speech and part of a syndrome of 'alogia'. There is currently no way of resolving the dispute between these two factions. Adherents of the latter view, however, do have to deal with one small matter, namely that if poverty of content of speech occurs in patients with poverty of speech, when exactly do they get the opportunity to be vague and convey little information, despite the number of words used?

3

The differential diagnosis of thought disorder

At times, thought disorder has been considered to be a symptom of, and only of, schizophrenia. Nowhere was this more true than in American psychiatry, which until comparatively recently laboured under Bleuler's (1911) dictate that it was one of the fundamental symptoms of schizophrenia. Harrow and Quinlan (1977), for example, noting that countless authors since Bleuler had 'affirmed its importance as a central feature of this disorder', stated that 'some astute clinicians have believed that reliance on disordered thinking is a certain way to distinguish schizophrenics from non-schizophrenics'. This view persisted until their own and others' studies (e.g. Harrow *et al.*, 1973; Harrow and Quinlan, 1977; Carlson and Goodwin, 1973; Taylor and Abrams, 1975) began to cast doubt on its universality in the disorder. These studies also made it clear, to nobody's surprise but their authors', that thought disorder was seen in at least one other disorder, mania.

This point was also made by Andreasen, in a typically pragmatic way, in one of her earliest studes (Andreasen *et al.*, 1974). She showed a group of forty-two psychiatrists, psychologists and social workers at the hospital where she worked six samples of prose and asked them to decide whether thought disorder was present and what diagnosis they suspected in each case. Two of the samples were from patients with schizophrenia, two from patients with mania, and the remaining two consisted of an extract from James Joyce's *Finnegans Wake* and part of a poem retyped in prose form, *The Perfection of Dentistry* by Marvin Bell. The hospital staff rated thought disorder as present more frequently in the manic patients than the schizophrenic patients. Half the sample thought it was also present in *The Perfection of Dentistry*, and *Finnegans Wake* received the highest ratings of all – forty of the forty-two staff considered that thought disorder was definitely present and twenty suspected a diagnosis of schizophrenia.

The fact that something bearing an at least passing resemblance to thought disorder can be seen in mania, and may be present in – or accessible to – some creative individuals, opens the door to the possibility that it is a quite widespread phenomenon. If mania, why not depression? Can it occur in normal individuals when they are not writing poetry or otherwise striving for creative expression?

Moving further afield, speech can certainly be rambling and incoherent in delirium, although when this happens it never seems to be referred to as thought disorder. Changes in the form of speech that are not completely dissimilar from the kind of abnormalities seen in schizophrenia have also been described in disorders as varied as epilepsy and autism.

Thought disorder in mania

In any textbook of psychiatry a statement will be found that disorders of thinking in mania take the form of distractibility and flight of ideas, where the train of thought is continually diverted by irrelevant associations; and that there may be clang associations, connections made on the basis of similarity of sound, rhymes or puns. Usually these accounts will also state that speech tends to be rapid and pressured, and they may mention that it can become severely incoherent in some cases.

Actual examples of manic thought disorder, however, are thin on the ground. One of the very few, and easily the finest, of these is a poem in Goodwin and Jamison's (1990) textbook on manic-depressive illness. This was written by a manic patient without pause over the course of a few minutes. Goodwin and Jamison felt its infectious cadence, tangential and occasionally loose language, frequent punning, fast and flowing rhythm and recurrent sexual reference captured many of the characteristic features of the hypomanic state.

God Is a Herbivore

Thyme passes, mixed with long grasses of herbs in the field.
Rosemary weeps into meadow sweeps
While curry is favored by the sun in its heaven.
The glinting scythe cuts the mustard twice
And the sage is ignored on its rock near the shore.
Hash is itself: high by being.
Laws says shallots shall not – so they shan't
    But. . .
The coriander meanders, the cumin seeds come
While a saffron canary eats juniper berry
Ignoring opened sesame seeds on the ground.

Hard data on manic thought disorder have been provided in a study by Carlson and Goodwin (1973). They followed twenty patients with well-diagnosed bipolar disorder through a manic episode. In the initial phase, which was observed in all twenty patients, there was increased activity, increased rate and initiation of speech, and mood changes characterised predominantly by euphoria, but also irritability and lability. The patients were overconfident, expansive and grandiose, showed increased sexual interest and activity, spent money inappropriately, smoked a lot, wrote letters and spent a lot of time on the telephone. The patients often described having racing thoughts, but objectively their thinking appeared coherent though sometimes going off on a tangent.

In the second stage, also observed in all twenty patients, pressure of speech and overactivity increased further. Mood progressed from predominant euphoria to increasing dysphoria and depression interspersed with explosive irritability and assaultative behaviour. Earlier paranoid and grandiose attitudes were now apparent as frank delusions. At this stage there was increasing disorganisation of thought and definite flight of ideas could be seen.

Fourteen of the twenty patients reached the final stage, characterised as a desperate panic-stricken and frequently hopeless state, often accompanied by frenzied activity. Delusions were bizarre and idiosyncratic; hallucinations could be present; and disorientation in time and place were sometimes seen. Thought processes that earlier had been only difficult to follow now became fragmented and confused. At this stage a definite loosening of associations was evident in many cases.

Thereafter improvement took place with the patients again passing through the second and the first stages. Over the whole course of the episode 100% of the patients showed pressure of speech, 100% showed extreme verbosity, 75% showed flight of ideas, 70% showed distractibility, and 70% were considered to have had loose associations.

The case to answer concerning thought disorder in mania is thus not whether it can occur – which, American views from the pre-DSM-III era to the contrary, has never been in doubt – but rather to what extent it is distinct from the equivalent symptom in schizophrenia. That the overlap can be great is easy to demonstrate. One of the spontaneous written productions used by Andreasen *et al.* (1974) in the study described above was from a patient whose illness was difficult to construe as anything other than schizophrenia. He had become progressively more withdrawn and reclusive since leaving school, was bizarre in appearance and behaviour, invented a language based on the anatomical structure of the throat and the binomial theorem, and showed flattening and inappropriateness of affect. However, what he wrote was in fact remarkably similar to the poem of Goodwin and Jamison's (1990) hypomanic patient:

Does water saunter? As to protein, might one tote-it-in? Is it a hydro-car-boat or a carbohydrate? As to any vitamin, might one invite-them-in? Is the dinner-all there with mineral? Is the bulk cellulose or the hulk swell-you-host? Might the medicine have met-us-some? Is it a platypus or adipose? Is the seasoning pleasing? Is food reserved to be preserved? Is one glad-to-give an additive?

Conversely, Durbin and Martin (1977) recorded the speech of six manic patients meeting the early (but strict) Feighner criteria for mania. One patient showed neologisms, referring to the Earth as the Moderator or Mother-ator, and a wall as an adjacentment. Another showed something that could easily be mistaken for poverty of content of speech. When answering a question about what his problems were, he replied:

In respect to them being problems, they have already been solved, however the solution of them is a problem, the passing them on is a problem and that is why I am here and actually, some of these solutions were acquired in my coming here and that's part of the reason I was here, and, the perfection of them came through here and the only problem now is the one we are solving now.

Wykes (1981) issued a challenge for the most radical view of all, that the whole concept of a distinction between schizophrenic and manic thought disorder might be nothing more than a convenient illusion. She obtained transcripts of thought-disordered speech from twelve acutely psychotic patients. On the basis of interview using the Present State Examination, plus review of case notes, eight of these had given a diagnosis of schizophrenia and four a diagnosis of mania. Nine psychiatrists were then asked to decide whether the patients were manic or schizophrenic on the basis of the transcripts alone. They were correct only 63% of the time for those with mania and only 46% of the time for those with schizophrenia.

Deciding whether manic and schizophrenic thought disorder are truly distinguishable would involve assessing thought disorder in as detailed a way as possible, under blind conditions, in large numbers of patients with rigorously diagnosed mania and schizophrenia. Andreasen (1979c) used the opportunity presented by the development of the TLC scale to do just this. She rated, blind to diagnosis, the speech of thirty-two manic and forty-five schizophrenic patients, matched for age and educational level. She later repeated the same exercise on a new sample of twenty-five manics and fifty schizophrenics (Andreasen and Grove, 1986b). The frequency with which the different items were rated as present (based on a rating of 2 or more, i.e. mild or greater) in each diagnostic group for the combined sample of patients is shown in Figure 3.1. The degree of overlap of the two forms of thought disorder was substantial: in both disorders every item that could be rated was rated, and those which were most frequent in schizophrenia also tended to be most frequent in mania. The core cluster of classical schizophrenic abnormalities, derailment, tangentiality, loss of goal and incoherence, and also illogicality, failed to distinguish the manic and schizophrenic statistically. Poverty of content of speech, however, was significantly more frequent in schizophrenia than mania, and two of the three abnormalities classically associated with mania, pressure of speech and distractible speech, were present at significantly higher rates in the manic patients. Circumstantiality was also over three times more common in mania. The very low rates of clang associations in both groups made it difficult to draw any conclusions concerning its differential affiliations.

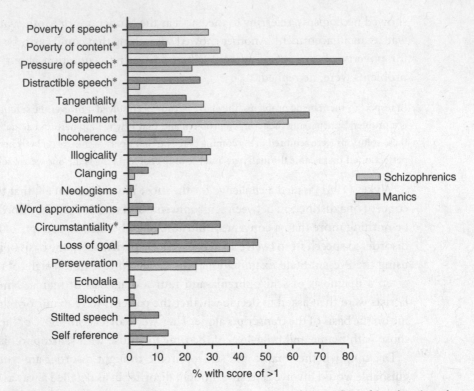

Figure 3.1   Frequencies of different TLC items in fifty-seven manic and ninety-five schizophrenic patients. Asterisks indicate significant differences (from Andreasen, 1979c; Andreasen and Grove 1986b).

When Andreasen went on to apply discriminant function analysis[1] to the data, however, the results were different. She included ten variables in the analysis: poverty of speech, poverty of content of speech, pressure of speech, distractible speech, tangentiality, derailment, incoherence, illogicality, loss of goal and perseveration. Despite the fact that many of the items had similar prevalences in the two groups of patients, the discriminant function correctly classified 95% of the schizophrenics and 69% of the manics in her 1979 sample. It also performed well when it was applied to the 1986 replication sample, correctly classifying 80% of the cases. Nearly all the discriminatory power derived from a small number of variables. Pressure of speech and distractible speech (associated with mania) accounted for over half the variance; derailment, poverty of content, loss of goal and poverty of speech (associated with schizophrenia) accounted for most of the

---

[1] A multivariate statistical technique which weights variables according to their alleged discriminatory power and then examines whether this leads to a bimodal or a unimodal distribution in a sample of individuals who exhibit the variables.

rest. Perseveration, tangentiality and incoherence and also illogicality were not discriminatory.

The somewhat surprising conclusion from these, and three further studies which had similar findings (Harvey *et al.*, 1984; Kufferle *et al.*, 1985; Oltmanns *et al.*, 1985), is that none of the currently recognised elements of thought disorder are the exclusive preserve of schizophrenia. Many of the features usually considered to be characteristic of schizophrenic thought disorder – including incoherence, illogicality, neologisms and word approximations – occur with more or less the same frequency in mania. A greater amount of poverty of content of speech in the former disorder and more pressure of speech and distractible speech in the latter, plus a slightly different admixture of other abnormalities may lend the two enough of a different flavour to be picked up by discriminant function analysis. But overall the similarities are more impressive than the differences.

One further abnormality which Andreasen found to be more characteristic of mania than schizophrenia is circumstantiality. Mentioned from time to time in descriptive accounts (Campbell, 1953; Lorenz, 1968) and found to be the most frequently rated abnormality after pressure of speech in one recent study (Taylor *et al.*, 1994), circumstantiality has become a largely forgotten element of manic speech. Nevertheless, manic or hypomanic patients are sometimes encountered whose speech is characterised partly or wholly by the inclusion of many tedious details and an endless succession of parenthetical remarks, as in the example shown in Box 3.1.

Box 3.1 Circumstantiality in a hypomanic patient

The patient is a fifty-one year-old woman with rapidly cycling bipolar disorder. She has not shown schizophrenic symptoms. She makes a full recovery between episodes, and her speech in particular becomes completely normal. There is no history of neurological disease, head injury or drug or alcohol abuse. While in a hypomanic episode she spoke in a measured way as follows:

Q   Tell me what it was that led you to come into hospital this time.

A   Um. . .Not being able to sleep. It actually started the day that I took up Henry's advice that I drink – I cut down on decaff as well as caffeinated coffee. I seem to remember, I think it was the Tuesday before I came in – I came in on the Saturday – and because at the hostel at the moment I am self-catering, which means I can go to Sainsbury's or the Co-op down the road, and you can buy table water, fizzy water at Sainsbury's for 21p or at the Co-op for 29p, and I was drinking that, and exotic fruit tea-bags, and I read a very interesting book, it's a best seller called "How to Heal your Life" by Louise – I can't remember the

Box 3.1 (cont.)

second name. It's about a woman who was diagnosed with vaginal cancer and that by sort of eating sensibly and the power of the mind – this is like a visualisation exercise which is also in the book – if you go to Cambridge Central Library, Lion Yard, you go past the general fiction and the music section is over there [gestures] and the kids' books are there [gestures] – and you have to visualise, say, your mother as a little child of three or four crying, and then you have to console her until she stops crying, and then you put her in your heart and keep her there.

And Louise whatever her name is also recommends that you ask your mother about her childhood, so that you could see she had a bad time and she was treating you badly because she was treated that way. But when I rang my mother, she said, 'Oh, I don't think you need anything like that, you've done enough in that respect.' But, like creative writing which is on my care plan to go to at the Bath House 2.30–4p.m. on Thursdays. It's taken by a white Irishman who is paid to take the group and he brings a big bag of books, poetry books and people can choose something to read if they want to and people bring their own poems to read.

Anyway, that's part of my care plan and it is very good and it works out very well because I go to word processing at 9.30 at Trumpington Street and I can type up whatever my poem is. And then Friday, it's voluntary work in the afternoons, and doing work at The White Hart in the evenings. And, also it's alternate Tuesdays now, the poetry group at CB1 which is run by a lady called Janet. She has been doing it since I was in B-ward and she – people go and have a drink. This is a funny story associated with this. She organises, what she was doing was having one, two, three first Tuesdays of the month with three poets who got paid out of the takings of everyone being there paying a pound each, and then the fourth one was, you'd bring your poem and read it aloud and then you'd get the pound back. And she's quite a showman, you know, she gets the show going and she gets people to be quiet and objects to people talking when she's talking, and she also organises an instrumental musician to play acoustic music. Do you want to hear this funny story?

Thought disorder in depression

In stark contrast to mania, nothing resembling incoherent speech is traditionally recognised in depression. The major abnormality described is a reduction of speech, which can vary from no more than a slight taciturnity to a state of almost complete muteness broken only by isolated whispered utterances. Beyond this, every psychiatrist will have noticed an additional disorder of the form of thinking, particularly in cases where there are psychotic symptoms. Thought appears narrowed and impoverished and in severe cases is reduced to a stereotyped litany of painful ruminations, which are produced almost immediately in response to questions on any topic. As Kraepelin (1913b) put it:

Their train of thought is orderly and connected, although mostly very monotonous; the patients always move in the same circle of ideas; on an attempt being made to divert them, they return again immediately to the old track. All mental activity is as a rule made difficult. The patients are absent-minded, forgetful, are easily tired, progress slowly or not all, and at the same time are sometimes most painfully precise in details.

Lewis (1934), who carried out one of the most authoritative clinical studies of depression, considered this account to be incomplete. He made a detailed clinical examination of sixty-one cases of 'melancholia', a term which in his hands corresponded closely to the modern concept of major depression. Twenty-two of the patients, rather than showing reduced speech, talked a great deal. Some continually requested interviews where they would speak at length and override any attempts to interrupt them or change the subject. Others talked whether or not there was anyone there to listen. Characteristically, the patients would apologise for their talkativeness, for taking up so much of the interviewer's time and making him write so much. The content of their speech was on the whole coherent, although it showed a great limitation in the number of topics, which revolved uniformly around depressive themes. However, a number of the patients showed something perhaps akin to distractibility, incorporating what other patients and staff said into their stream of talk, repeating it, applying it to themselves or even punning on it. Some examples of the abnormalities Lewis described are shown in Box 3.2

Box 3.2 Lewis on speech in depression

(From Lewis, 1934)

M.B. and J.G. kept repeating the remarks of other patients and applying them to themselves, with a running commentary, or dealing in a similar way with remarks addressed to them by the doctors or nurses, which they repeated, distorted, commented on and played with, even making puns, but always in the sense of self-reproach, etc. They commented on their own behaviour, e.g., 'I was talking all night. I'm like a clock; I stop for a while and then I start again.' 'I came here for talking.' 'I'm more troubled than the others that keep getting out of bed. I stay in bed.' They would both stop if requested, but only for a few minutes.

H.C. whimpered all the time; occasionally she would utter a sharp comment or rebuke, but most of her almost inaudible talk was in the nature of comment on herself and those around her.

Box 3.2 (cont.)

A.F., however, was different. Importunate, with very few topics, she beset all the nurses and doctors whom she saw with inquiries, requests for reassurance and complaints, without paying any heed to suitability of time and place. Left to herself, she became silent.

Among the younger women of this group, importunity was striking, with the exception of E.B., who, during one period of her illness, talked constantly about her own behaviour and that of the other patients in a low, scarcely audible voice, much like the three older women mentioned above. She continued with this even when there was no audience. At an earlier stage she had talked profusely, but only when addressed.

J.C. called one, whenever one appeared, to draw attention to her pains and discomforts. If no one was near her, except other patients, she remained silent. She would continue talking so that one had difficulty in getting away from her bedside. She repeated the same set of phrases over and over, as did also L.C., who would call out 'May I stay here, may I stay here' hundreds of times in a day, i.e., as often as a nurse or a doctor walked by her bed. D.N. remained quiet until someone came near her; she would then call out, and if it were the doctor ask for a private interview; during such interviews she would talk at great speed, running over the same ground in almost the same words, often refusing to leave the room when the interview was over, but persisting with her old requests for reassurance and her protestations.

G.S. talked incessantly, audience or no audience, on a few topics with verbal reiteration, mostly in a loud, whining voice, with a formal precision of phrase, like a school-mistress.

E.B., just referred to, repeated over and over the same two or three phrases in a rather loud voice, with much whining and tearless sobbing. She would not, during this period, answer questions relevantly unless they bore on the burden of her complaint.

L.H. was incessantly proclaiming her difficulties and wrongs, protesting against unjust accusations. She would do this in a loud voice until midnight sometimes; she would follow one about in the ward, demanding reassurance or promises, and she did not talk if there was no audience. She would converse only on these few topics.

I.M. was continually asking for interviews, at which she reiterated the same few complaints, and at the end of which she was most reluctant to leave the room, going on with her declarations of unhappiness, headache, etc. She did not talk unless she had an audience. She would stop, moreover, if interrupted, and it was possible to carry on a conversation with her and to direct its course.

There are only two men who talked a lot. One, A.H., was continually asking for an interview, and harped on a few topics – his wickedness and his ill-health – but he did not talk much to the other patients or to the nurses, and his conversation could be deflected.

The other loquacious man, R.H., railed loudly and vehemently about his misery, hopelessness, cowardice. In him alone, however, hypomanic features might be recognized: he surrounded himself with books, which he read rapidly; he waved his arms when talking and otherwise gesticulated; he gave the impression of gusto, of enjoying his tirades against himself and fate.

Ianzito *et al.* (1974) purported to find considerably more evidence of thought disorder in severe depression. From a sample of 200 patients admitted to hospital over a six-month period they isolated a group of forty-seven who met their own diagnostic criteria for affective disorder, depressed type. Patients who fulfilled criteria for bipolar disorder were excluded, as were any who had additional diagnoses, such as alcoholism, sociopathy or organic brain disease. The patients were also followed up eighteen months later to confirm that no other disorder had appeared in the interim. Six of the forty-seven patients (13%) were rated as showing mild thought disorder, which in their rating scheme included circumstantiality and vagueness; seven (15%) showed moderate thought disorder, as indicated by paralogical (see Chapter 4) or unrelated responses, tangentiality or flight of ideas; and two (4%) were rated as having severe thought disorder, showing one or more of the features of neologisms, echolalia, perseveration, clang associations or word salad. The overall rate of thought disorder was approximately a third of that seen in a comparison group of thirty-four patients with a diagnosis of acute schizophrenia.

Andreasen (1979c) also included a group of thirty-six depressed patients in her original validation study of the TLC scale. The frequency of scores of 2 or greater are shown in Figure 3.2, where they are compared with the rates for ninety-four normal subjects from the study of Andreasen and Grove (1986b). In general, the scores on most subtypes of thought disorder were low, and many of the patients did not rate on them at all. As expected, they showed a significantly increased frequency of poverty of speech compared with the normal subjects. More unexpectedly, but by no means counter-intuitively, they also showed an elevated rate of poverty of content of speech. As remarked on by Kraepelin (1913b), there was also an increased rate of circumstantiality. At 11%, self-referential speech was also relatively frequent, perhaps reflecting the depressed patient's tendency to divert any topic of conversation back to a small circle of depressive ideas. Derailment and loss of goal were present no more freqently than in the normal subjects. Incoherence, neologisms, word approximations and illogicality were not seen. The depressed patients did, however, show a higher frequency of tangentiality than normal subjects.

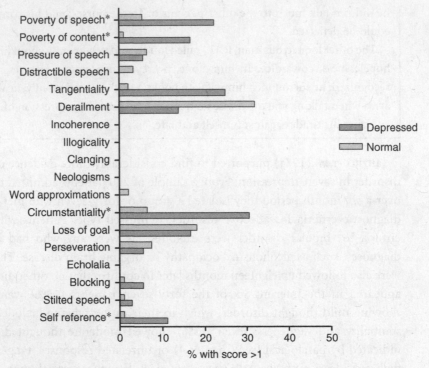

Figure 3.2   Frequencies of different TLC scale items in thirty-six depressed patients and ninety-four normal individuals. Asterisks indicate significantly higher rates in the patients (from Andreasen, 1979c; Andreasen and Grove 1986b).

Ianzito et al.'s study appears to suggest that thought disorder which is essentially similar in nature to that seen in schizophrenia occurs with appreciable frequency in patients with depression. In contrast, Andreasen's (1979c) findings paint a more sober and conventional picture. Her conclusion was that thought disorder is infrequent in depression, tends to be mild when it does occur, and its profile of poverty of speech, poverty of content of speech and circumstantiality is both different to that of schizophrenia and consistent with the known features of depression. There are certainly reasons to be cautious in accepting Ianzito et al.'s findings at face value: at 56% the frequency of thought disorder in their schizo-phrenic sample was high. Additionally, at least a quarter of their depressed patients were psychotic and they stated that 'many showed such typical "schizophrenic" experiences as depersonalization, thought withdrawal, and audible thoughts'. One explanation of their high rate and schizophrenia-like character of thought disorder might be that they included a number of misdiagnosed schizophrenic or schizoaf-fective patients. Another, however, could be that when depression becomes severe enough to be designated psychotic depression, thought disorder enters the clinical picture along with all the other symptoms which make the differential diagnosis of schizophrenia and affective disorder more than a trivially easy exercise.

Delirium

Delirium is currently the most widely used term to describe the acute disturbance of brain function which can be produced by any number of pathological processes, from head injury to anoxia to metabolic disturbances to the toxic effects of drugs. Incoherence of speech is not an invariable part of the picture – its only essential feature is confusion, which is always present to some degree – but along with visual hallucinations it is seen frequently enough to make it one of the three hallmark symptoms of the syndrome.

The rambling speech of delirium is easy to recognise, but what makes it so is more difficult to define. Thinking certainly appears to be disorganised in its own right, becoming disjointed, fragmented and chaotic, and in extreme cases reduced to incoherent muttering. At the same time, most authors (e.g. Lipowski, 1990; Lishman, 1998; Caraceni and Grassi, 2003) agree that several other processes are also at work. One of the most striking of these is the intrusion of vivid and bizarre dream-like thoughts and images into consciousness, which then become woven into the stream of thought. Perhaps because the patient is always ill and usually in hospital, these often revolve around themes of danger, disability, mutilation and death.

A disorder of attention also seems to be involved: patients have difficulty in focusing their thoughts or formulating complex ideas, and a sustained directed train of thought is difficult to maintain. Speech is replete with logical contradictions which go unappreciated – the patient may address the interviewer as 'Doctor' but then deny knowledge of his or her occupation. Distractibility and perseveration may be present. Thinking is also noticeably concrete and literal, and the content tends to be banal and impoverished. Thought may be slowed down or speeded up; the patient may be mute, or at the other extreme there may be a ceaseless flow of speech, often with repetition of the same words and themes.

Such a description appears to set the incoherent speech of delirium apart from that seen in schizophrenia, but is this really the case? One of the few psychiatrists to pose this question, and the only one to then go on to do a study to answer it, is Cutting.[2] He (Cutting, 1987; see also Cutting, 1980) examined seventy-four patients who showed psychosis in the setting of some clearly identifiable organic cause. Confusion was present at the time of examination in sixty-two (84%) of the patients and most of the rest had shown cognitive impairment at some point.

---

[2] Cutting is an individualistic British psychiatrist and writer who has tackled many outstanding questions in psychosis, clinical, diagnostic, psychological and, most recently, philosophical.

Table 3.1 Frequencies of different TLC items in delirious and schizophrenic patients
(From Cutting, 1987, reproduced with permission)

TLC item	Delirium ($N = 74$)	Schizophrenia ($N = 74$)
Poverty of speech	14	1
Poverty of content	1	1
Pressure of speech	2	0
Distractible speech	2	0
Tangentiality	6	2
Derailment	0	10
Incoherence	1	3
Illogicality	15	0
Clanging	0	0
Neologisms	0	1
Word approximations	2	0
Circumstantiality	4	1
Loss of goal	0	1
Perseveration	0	0
Echolalia	0	0
Blocking	0	1
Stilted speech	0	2
Self reference	0	0

Note: The patients were rated according to the presence of the most predominant form of marked abnormality, and so the scoring is not comparable with that used in Andreasen's studies.

Cutting interviewed each patient using the Present State Examination, and rated their speech using the TLC scale.

Thought disorder was present in forty-seven of the seventy-four patients (63%). A full breakdown of the TLC ratings is shown in Table 3.1, together with those for a comparison group of seventy-four patients with acute schizophrenia. The most frequent abnormality was illogicality, which was present in fifteen patients (20%). Cutting considered, however, that this designation did not fully capture the quality of the abnormality, which always took the form of giving absurd answers to questions about orientation, and facile and inconsequential explanations for these (he suggested the term fantastic disorientation instead). For example, one patient claimed that it must be the 20 May because her sister had died then, without explaining why the date of her sister's death should determine today's date. Other patients gave answers to questions about their location which included: East Finchley airport, waiting at a bus-stop, on a boat, in Wales (and then a minute later in London). Such replies could not be attributed simply to memory impairment or perceptual disorder because of the bizarre choice of place – there is no airport in East Finchley – and because of the equally bizarre explanations given, such as 'Well, it looks a bit like an airport' or 'It's a boat because all my friends are here.' One patient, who believed he was at home, could not understand why his wife had bought so many beds.

Fourteen patients (19%) showed poverty of speech. This typically took the form of a combination of apathy, slow speech and restricted or impoverished output; often the patients only responded monosyllabically.

Six patients (8%) showed tangentiality. This took the form of intermittently irrelevant comments occurring in the course of an otherwise fairly lucid conversation. As with illogicality, Cutting felt that the patients' replies went beyond the normal usage of the term, being completely unrelated to the question rather than showing the subtle or oblique relationship implied by Andreasen's definition. Thus one patient, when asked where he was, replied that he was allergic to flowers. Another replied to a question about orientation by saying, 'You're nervous of people, I can see that.'

Among the remaining patients, four had prominent circumstantiality, giving long rambling accounts. One patient showed poverty of content of speech. Two patients showed distractibility, interrupting their flow of talk every time there was a noise. Pressure of speech was present in two patients, who both also showed flight of ideas. Incoherence was rated as present only in one patient who mumbled ungrammatically. Derailment and loss of goal were conspicuous by their absence. Surprisingly, perseveration was not seen in any of the patients.

Only two patients in Cutting's (1987) study showed unusual use of words. One referred to a female junior doctor as a doctoress, and the other believed, as part of a complex persecutory delusion, that he had a parallel circulatory system which he called 'man's money'. While this mirrors the widely held view that language disorder is uncommon in delirium (Chédru and Geschwind, 1972; Kitselman, 1981), or usually reflects non-linguistic disturbances (Caraceni and Grassi, 2003), occasional patients in whom this is prominent have been described. In such cases delirious speech can be very reminiscent of thought-disordered schizophrenia. In the first report of this phenomenon, Curran and Schilder[3] (1935) described three acutely confused patients who showed dysphasic-type misnamings and circumlocutions (Cigarette – 'cigaroot'; eyes – 'glimmers'; thumb – 'small hand'; 'I got no furniture on', referring to clothes). They were all excited and overtalkative and, as they improved, they also showed a queer sort of flightiness and circumstantiality. When asked what kind of a place he was in, one replied, 'This here's supposed to be like a straightening out place, a place that is really down and out.' Another replied

---

[3] Schilder was a German psychiatrist who had done influential work on thought disorder before emigrating to America to become director of Bellevue Hospital, New York.

to a question about whether he was talking in a sensible way with, 'In conversation with any person I should say, I should imagine, I should say I am talking plenty sense. The individual with whom I am contraversing, I am trying to come to an agreement with the individual to give him the benefit of my conversation and to really have an impression in his own mind that my conversation is given in the way it was all the time.'

Weinstein and Kahn (1952) made similar observations in a group of patients with 'altered behavior in association with intracranial disease'. Their patients showed multiple misnamings of objects, plus neologisms and obscure metaphorical phrases in the setting of speech which did not show other features of dysphasia – their words were not garbled, the rhythm of speech was normal and there was no perseveration. Later Clarke *et al.* (1958) gave a detailed description of a patient with Wernicke's encephalopathy, in whom, as they put it, the speech disorder appeared to transcend ordinary dysphasia and involved an underlying derangement of thought. This is summarised in Box 3.3.

Box 3.3 Language disorder in a patient with Wernicke's encephalopathy

(From Clarke *et al.*, 1958)

The patient was a 62-year-old man with a long history of alcoholism. One week before admission he had become sleepy and his mind had begun to wander – he talked of the past and claimed to have seen long dead relatives. He also complained of double vision, weakness in the legs and numbness and coldness in the fingers of both hands.

On examination he was facile, euphoric and disoriented, believing that he was in a flat near the hospital and that the other patients were railway workers. Memory for recent events was virtually nonexistent and he confabulated freely. Neurological examination revealed unequal pupils, nystagmus and impaired conjugate gaze in all directions.

During the earlier stages of his illness, the patient showed a curious language disorder which was most apparent when he was asked to name objects, define words, explain proverbs, etc. He named a cigarette lighter as a 'top hat lighter; asphalts and all that – tobacco accessory'; a penknife as a 'smoke affair – smoke button'; and a spanner as a 'poetic collector'. A striking feature of his speech was his tendency to use long and unusual words in quite inappropriate ways. Thus he referred to an interview as a 'psychoanalogical categoreal examination' and gave as his reason for being in hospital that he was 'suffering from expectorations of cholera attacks'. Occasionally, frank neologisms appeared in his speech, e.g. 'cosmey' to denote a variety of wood and 'stanch' to denote a meal.

Perseveration of both words and ideas was frequent, but more striking was the patient's flightiness, exuberance, and a certain queer circumstantiality. Any task involving directed thinking provoked a long, discursive, and often totally incoherent flood of speech. For example when asked to explain the idiom *Safety first*, he replied: 'It's an idea to make sure during any accident that is taking place. Light for the patient. First claim is made as the duty of the instruments used to make sure that the method is going to give you the results – perfect patient.' His interpretation of *Too many cooks spoil the broth* was: 'Too many cooks spoil the broth. I'm good enough to do the cooking without your assistance. Just a plain statement that goes out from the ordinary cook. An antagonistic outlook they've got on the affiliated amount of medical experience they possess.'

A curious pedantry was also evident at times. For example he named a rubber as 'an india rubber or as you say in more obvious language an india rubber eraser', and defined a corkscrew as 'an automatic accessory for bunging beers out of bottles'.

Grammar and syntax were formally correct.

He was treated with thiamine and improved over several weeks. Four months after admission he was well enough to be discharged to another institution, but showed dense amnesia and confabulation. A further 16 months later he was found to be approximately oriented in time, place and person. Although his memory was still grossly impaired for recent events and events for up to 5–10 years prior to the onset of illness he was no longer confabulated. The patient's conversation was lucid and fluent and he was considered to show minimal language abnormality; however, he still gave some paraphasic and otherwise inappropriate responses when explaining idioms and proverbs.

The thought disorder associated with delirium thus seems in the main to be only a crude copy of its counterpart in functional psychosis. Occasionally, though, it can resemble schizophrenic speech closely enough to give one pause for thought. When it does, presence of language abnormality appears to be a crucial factor in conferring the similarity. This may have implications for the nature of schizophrenic thought disorder itself, a point which is returned to in Chapter 4.

Epilepsy

People with epilepsy have had to endure many prejudices, one of which has been the claim that they show a characteristic personality type. In the past, the traits subsumed under the term 'epileptic personality' included, but were not limited to: egocentricity, ponderousness, pedantry, slowness, religiosity, devoutness, goodheartedness, sincerity, obsequiousness, piety, thrift, conscientiousness, moral rectitude, humourlessness, sanctimoniousness, bigotry, hypocrisy, untrustworthiness, slyness, two-facedness, spitefulness, vengefulness, viciousness, explosiveness and brutality. Some of these frequently contradictory epithets are recognisable as nothing more than the kind of thoughtless caricaturing of patients that was once fashionable among psychiatrists working in asylums, where many patients with epilepsy were forced to spend their days. Others seem to be altogether too characteristic of the human condition to be attributable to the effects of neurological disease. But it is possible that a small minority of the above terms reflect a more well-founded claim that there is a specific personality syndrome associated with epilepsy, one of the major features of which is an alteration in the form of thinking.

According to Blumer (1975, 1995), the principal contemporary apologist for this view, Kraepelin (1923) gave one of the first balanced accounts of certain changes which gradually developed in more than half of the epileptic patients 'coming to the attention of the psychiatrist'. These took the form of a slowing and meticulousness of mental processes, which resulted in a peculiar circumstantiality. Accompanying this could be emotional changes, including lability of mood and religiosity, but above all irritability. Thinking could become impoverished and memory sometimes suffered in advanced cases.

This slowness, circumstantiality and painstaking quality of thought in epileptic patients, often referred to as 'viscosity' or 'adhesiveness', was described again and again by authors of this period. It was captured particularly eloquently by Gruhle (1930) (quoted by Blumer, 1995):

He is enormously circumstantial, it takes him a long time to get to the point, he uses expletives as well as an excessive number of polite expressions, fills in with quotations, and tries to insure himself in advance against any possible misunderstanding.

After a lull during which the psychiatric aspects of epilepsy were largely ignored, the concept of epileptic personality was revived, this time as a syndrome associated with temporal lobe epilepsy. Central to this revival was a series of studies carried out by Gastaut and his co-workers (Gastaut *et al.*, 1953; Gastaut, 1954; Gastaut and Collomb, 1954) on patients whose epilepsy was well-characterised, clinically and electroencephalographically. They observed that patients with temporal lobe epilepsy, plus a small number of those with secondary generalised epilepsy,[4] but

---

[4] Secondary generalised epilepsy, also known as the Lennox–Gastaut syndrome, refers to a form of generalised seizures seen in patients with diffuse brain damage from any cause, which is often difficult to control.

not those with other forms of epilepsy, showed mental slowness and impulsive behaviour. They also documented hyposexuality for the first time in this group of patients.

Combining these features with some of the emotional changes described in earlier accounts, Blumer (Blumer, 1975; Blumer and Benson, 1975), Bear (Bear and Fedio, Bear, 1979) and Geschwind (Waxman and Geschwind, 1975; Geschwind, 1979) reached a consensus on the features of a stable personality syndrome, which occurred in patients with temporal lobe epilepsy strikingly more than in other forms of epilepsy, and which tended to develop approximately two years after the onset of seizures. The three components of this syndrome were: (i) a form of circumstantiality with additional features of viscosity or adhesiveness of thought, and sometimes also associated with hypergraphia, excessive and detailed writing; (ii) hyposexuality, sometimes associated with sexual deviations, or rarely hypersexuality; and (iii) emotional changes including lability of mood, irritability, dysphoria, anxiety and paranoid attitudes, as well as more nebulous constructs embodied by terms like 'spirituality', 'deepened emotional life' and 'increased sense of personal destiny'.

If clinical impression is anything to go by, the existence of such a syndrome is undeniable. Blumer and Benson (1975) gave the example of a fifty-three-year-old man who underwent a right temporal lobectomy for epilepsy at the age of forty. Prior to the operation he had been irritable and moody for days at a time. He had married for companionship and he and his wife had sex only a few times during the first eight years of the marriage and never thereafter. After surgery, his moodiness gradually subsided and he enthusiastically participated in a number of community and church activities. He was both verbose and meticulous in his statements. For example, when asked what he would do if he saw a fire in a theatre, or if he found a stamped envelope in the street, he gave traditional answers but made sure that all possibilities were covered; for instance, he considered whether or not the stamp was cancelled and whether the fire was large or small, had just begun, or had been going for some time. He sent his doctor regular reports on daily events, including his dreams. Characteristic of these communications was the squirrel story, which is reproduced in Box 3.4.

In order to validate the temporal lobe personality syndrome, Bear and Fedio (1977) devised a 100-item questionnaire consisting of true or false questions directed to eighteen of its proposed features. These covered emotionality, altered sexual interest, circumstantiality, viscosity of thought, hypermoralism, sense of personal destiny, hypergraphia, religiosity, philosophical interest, and also elation/ euphoria, sadness, anger, aggression, guilt, obsessionalism, paranoia, humourlessness and sobriety. They administered this to twenty-seven patients with temporal lobe epilepsy and to two control groups, one consisting of twelve normal adults of

Box 3.4 The squirrel story: circumstantiality and deepened emotion in a patient with temporal lobe epilepsy

(From Blumer and Benson, 1975, reproduced with permission)

When we moved from an upstairs apartment to a first floor one (Dec. 1, 19–), the squirrels I feed night and morning followed right with us. The squirrels are very tame and cute. They would feed out of my wife's and my hands. While I watch the door for a man to pick her up for work while she got ready I would prop the screen door open about 4 inches and feed them from inside by opening the inside door about an inch. They would come through the screen door opening and feed as I gave them food through the crack in the inside door. They would sit on the door sill and eat it (most of the time). It was winter and this way I could feed them while inside. When I went walking I would prop the screen door open and place some food in a dish on the door sill and they would feed from that. One day I did not put the dish there, they had enough, and went walking. When I came back the screen door had not gone completely shut and they had chewed about one third of the door away. I repaired this with water putty and painted it. Then to teach them to stay away from it I rubbed some Red Pepper on the repair with my finger. As I watched the next day one of them must have got into it. He just stood on the porch. You could see he was in awful pain, he quivered, cried and dripped from the mouth. It was awful to witness but they have not bothered the door since. The next day (June 5) I took a dish of peanuts out on the porch to feed them. They all acted normal until I saw one coming from the side to get in the dish. He upset it and I went to brush him away with my hand. As I did he gave me a good bite on the outside of the right hand at the little finger. I washed it good with soap and water and put on some Merthiolate. I have been taught to watch the animal. If it has Rabies it will die in 10 to 14 days giving time to start the Pasteur treatment. Also the further from the head the bite is the longer it takes. Rabies is a virus of the nerves following the nerves from the bite to the head where it is fatal.

Our squirrels are fed clean food and water. They do not get into any dead or rotten food. They all are as healthy as can be. Have a pretty coat and the cutest habits you would want to see. The litter they had this spring were the most domesticated I have ever seen. *Wouldn't you fight anything you knew treated you like he was with red pepper?* Squirrels are like other forms of life. One alone you can train and it will respond without any trouble. But when another one or two show on the scene they are always fighting each other and chasing each other from the source of food. Also one always wants to be a bully. You should hear them growl and chase each other away when more than one tries to feed from the same dish.

I was a little alarmed about the bite because we have some neighbors who are scared of any animal at all. All they can say is 'you know they can give you Rabies'. Knowing circumstances I managed to conquer my nerves for a month and the squirrel was here and healthy as ever. After 2 weeks I felt safe, free and my nerves were quiet again ... August 12 a squirrel came to the door. I thought it was a meek one. I held a piece of Graham Cracker toward it. It looked at me and went for my hand as if to take the cracker. It ignored the cracker and bit my finger instead. This time it was the little finger of the left hand. Within 10 seconds the bottom of my stomach hurt, I got a headache and the base of my throat started to hurt and feel tight. As I write this it is bringing back memories and I can feel it again.

I stood it as long as I possibly could. The worry was making a wreck of me. Then I went to Dr. R. August 17. He is treating me as you did. Reassuring me it was my nerves. Proving my thoughts and worries wrong and in my own thoughts. He told me to increase my Valium to half a tablet at 8:00 a.m. and half at 4:00 p.m. He also told me something I had read and forgot. The state is considered Rabies free. There has not been a case I think he said in 5 or 7 years. This program of having dogs injected to prevent Rabies is purely political to make money and keep a record of dogs for licensing. Now I remember reading that in the paper when they started the program a few years ago.

Also do not feed the squirrels by hand. Toss the food to them or put it on a plate for them. They are wild animals and while no Rabies has been reported for a long time they can chew you up bad then infection maybe. He also reminded me that Bats are the ones that are full of Rabies. This I knew from childhood. Now I feed the squirrels in a dish on the porch. *No more by hand.* I slowly got ahold of myself again.

comparable age, education and social level, and the other made up of nine patients with neuromuscular diseases. The subjects completed a self-rated version of the questionnaire, and someone who knew them well completed an observer-rated version. The temporal lobe epilepsy patients were found to have significantly higher overall scores than the two control groups on both versions of the scale. All eighteen traits distinguished the epileptic patients from the controls on the self-rated scale, and fourteen of them also did so on the observer-rated scale. Circumstantiality and viscosity of thought were among the individual items showing the most marked differences. Emotionality and religiousness also discriminated the groups well. There were, however, only small differences between the epileptic patients and the two control groups for hypergraphia and altered sexuality.

Bear and Fedio concluded that a 'consistent profile of changes in behaviour (obsessionalism, circumstantiality), thought (religious and philosophical interest), and affect (anger, emotionality, and sadness) thus appears to be the specific consequence of a temporal epileptic focus.' But this conclusion was not yet warranted. There was the small matter of establishing that the syndrome was not equally a feature of other types of epilepsy. Additionally, as Lishman (1998) pointed out, slowing, ponderousness and perseverativeness, not to mention irritability, poor impulse control and emotional lability are the hallmarks of many forms of brain damage, and for a wide range of reasons brain damage is a common accompaniment of epilepsy.[5]

The results of the six further studies using the Bear–Fedio inventory are summarised in Table 3.2. A common feature of these studies is their small sample size, but their results are highly consistent. They all support Bear and Fedio's original finding that patients with temporal lobe epilepsy score significantly more highly than normal individuals. However, they are nearly as uniform in failing to find differences between patients with temporal lobe and other forms of epilepsy. Even in the one study which found clearly higher scores on a modified form of the Bear–Fedio Inventory in temporal lobe epilepsy patients compared with those with generalised epilepsy (Bear *et al.*, 1982), only four out of fourteen traits (religiosity, philosophical interests, sadness and emotionality) significantly discriminated the groups.

Only one of these studies addressed the confounding issue of brain damage. Mungas (1982) compared scores on the Bear–Fedio Inventory in nineteen patients with temporal lobe epilepsy and a group of fourteen patients with brain damage from a variety of causes. These latter patients were perhaps not the ideal control group, since four were violent, one abused drugs, one had Huntington's disease and at least four had psychiatric histories. At any rate, there were no significant differences between the groups on either the self-rated or observer-rated versions of the scale.

The available evidence certainly supports the clinical impression that some patients with epilepsy show circumstantiality, and possibly a unique form of circumstantially at that. This, however, is not exclusive to temporal lobe epilepsy. Nor is it ruled out that it is due to the co-existing brain damage that is commonly present in patients with epilepsy, rather than the epilepsy itself – the definitive study would require a considerably less wayward brain-damaged group than the one Mungas (1982) used. Furthermore, while there is no real doubt that the epileptic personality syndrome can develop in patients who do not have a diagnosis of psychosis (Blumer, 1995), how much of it is due to co-existing psychiatric

---

[5] Brain damage may be the cause of a patient's seizures, or be acquired as a result of having seizures, for example through repeated head trauma, anoxia and the shadowy concept of epileptic dementia.

Table 3.2 Studies comparing scores on the Bear-Fedio Inventory between temporal lobe epilepsy patients and other groups

Study	Samples	Self-rated scale	Observer-rated scale	Comment
TLE vs. normal subjects				
Master et al. (1984)	55 TLE 40 volunteers	Higher	Higher	
Rodin and Schmaltz (1984)	36 TLE 40 hospital employees	Higher	—	
Brandt et al. (1985)	47 TLE 14 volunteers	Higher	—	
TLE vs. other epilepsy				
Hermann and Riel (1981)	14 TLE 14 GE	NSD	Higher	TLE patients had significantly higher scores in 4 of 18 categories
Bear et al.(1982)	10 TLE 10 GE/other focal epilepsy	—	Higher	Used modified form of observer-rated scale, with ratings made by clinicians. Both groups had psychiatric histories
Master et al. (1984)	55 TLE 16 GE	NSD	NSD	
Rodin and Schmaltz (1984)	36 temporal spike foci 33 diffuse spike-and-wave	?		Patients with temporal foci nonsignificantly higher in 13 of 18 categories
Brandt et al (1985)	47 TLE 10 GE	NSD	NSD	
TLE vs. other brain disease				
Mungas (1982)	14 TLE 13 brain disease	NSD	NSD	Brain disease patients also had 'behavioural problems'

Notes: TLE – temporal lobe epilepsy.
GE – generalised epilepsy.

morbidity is difficult to ascertain – several of the above studies (Mungas, 1981; Bear et al., 1982; Master et al., 1984) have found that unselected groups of psychiatric patients show a not-dissimilar profile of scores on the Bear–Fedio Inventory to that seen in epileptic patients.

Autism and Asperger's syndrome

Approximately half of all patients with autism never acquire useful speech, and in those who do it develops abnormally. Some of these latter patients retain the typical autistic features of echolalia, reversal of pronouns, and use of stereotyped and idiosyncratic words and phrases into adult life, but in others speech becomes grammatically normal and many autistic adults have a large vocabulary. Even in these so-called high functioning patients, however, and in those with the milder but otherwise essentially similar disorder of Asperger's syndrome, who typically have a full command of language, speech is almost always noticeably odd.

To psychologists and psychiatrists working in the field of autism, much of this abnormality is understandable as part of the wider impairment of reciprocal social interaction that is one of the core features of the disorder. Autistic and Asperger patients do not use speech in the service of social interaction, and fail to observe the niceties of polite conversation. As Wing[6] (Wing, 1981, 1996; Wing and Attwood, 1987) has put it, they talk at people rather than to them, immediately begin asking multiple questions without the usual conversational openers, ignore the normal rules of turn-taking and speak at length on topics which are of interest only to them. On being asked a question about why police were needed, one patient launched into a history of the police beginning with Sir Robert Peel.

The case of Peter (actually a composite of several real cases), described by Frith (2003) illustrates several of these features:

He was not at all shy and often approached visitors to the house or the school, asking their names and addresses. 'Dulwich', he would say, 'that is number 12.' Next time they came, the same interchange would take place. Although he was often rather too talkative, in a repetitive sort of way ('Today is Monday, yesterday was Sunday, tomorrow is Tuesday and we are going to visit Grandma'), it was often strangely difficult to get important information from him. For instance, when he was quite badly injured after a fall, he never told anyone about it, and his mother was horrified when she discovered blood on his clothes as she put them in the washing machine. Peter's understanding was extremely literal. Once, when his mother remarked that his sister had been crying her eyes out, he anxiously looked on the floor to see if the eyes were there. However, he studiously learned the meaning of such 'silly phrases', and was keen to use them himself, even when not entirely appropriate.

[6] Lorna Wing, married to J. K. Wing of Chapters 1 and 2.

Not all the features of the speech of autistic and Asperger patients are easy to explain on this basis. Some patients speak very little, despite having good speech (Wing, 1996). Many have a fascination with long words and use pedantic turns of phrase. One of Wing and Attwood's (1987) patients, a boy, said, 'I wish to thank you for the hospitality you have extended to me this afternoon', in response to being given a cup of tea. Frith (2003) described an adult patient who always announced himself by saying, 'This is M. C. Smith, your nephew, speaking', when he telephoned his favourite aunt. Another patient referred to a hole in his sock as 'a temporary loss of knitting' (Wing, 1981). Sometimes there are stereotyped repetitions of words and phrases like 'more or less' or 'I caused a lot of trouble, didn't I?' (Simmons and Baltaxe, 1975). Some patients ask the same questions over and over again, regardless of the answers they receive. Occasionally, neologisms and idiosyncratic words are used. For example, Tantam (1991) described a patient with Asperger's syndrome who believed that he was in a 'missage' (asleep) between two 'boating lines' (periods of existence).

In such circumstances a study using the TLC in autism is in order. Rumsey *et al.* (1986) recruited a sample of fourteen adult patients who met DSM III criteria for autism, or autism residual state.[7] None of the patients had epilepsy or other neurological disorders, and most were of normal IQ (two had IQs in the mentally handicapped range and three showed verbal IQs in the handicapped range coupled with normal or superior performance IQs). Interviews, in which the patients first had to read out a short passage of prose, then talk freely about themselves, and finally answer questions on various topics, were videotaped and later rated by Andreasen. Her TLC ratings are shown in Figure 3.3, along with those for a group of age-matched normal controls. The most frequently rated item was poverty of speech, which was present in ten of the patients (71%). These included one patient who was mute, another who had minimal speech, and one patient who showed telegraphic speech. Seven patients (50%) were rated on poverty of content of speech. Perseveration was present in eight patients (57%). These were the only items that were significantly more frequent than in the normal subjects. However, three of the patients scored on echolalia, three on incoherence and two on tangentiality; this was in contrast to none of the control group.

Rumsey *et al.* (1986) commented that the high ratings they found on perseveration and low ratings on loss of goal were likely to reflect austic single-mindedness and rigidity – rather than modifying the direction of their conversation in response to the normal give and take of the interview, the patients tended to adhere rigidly to a topic and resist any attempt to shift them from it. It is also possible that the

---

[7] Seven of the patients had in fact been diagnosed by Kanner.

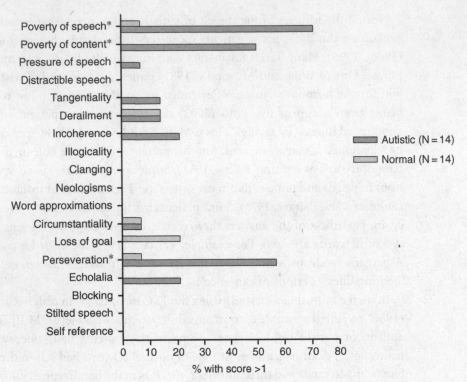

Figure 3.3   Frequencies of different TLC items in fourteen adult autistic patients and fourteen normal individuals. Asterisks indicate significantly higher rates in the patients (from Rumsey *et al.*, 1986).

poverty of content of speech they found could to some extent reflect the repetitiveness of autistic speech.

Further information on autistic speech comes from a quite different source. From the 1960s a group of disorders where language fails to develop normally, but not in the setting of a general pattern of developmental impairment, began to be described and categorised. Originally known as developmental dysphasias and now known as specific language impairments, their classification is still a matter of debate (e.g. Rapin and Allen, 1983; Bishop and Rosenbloom, 1987), but they are agreed to fall into three broad categories. Some children show comprehension deficits and these necessarily also give rise to problems with expression. Others show impaired expression despite good comprehension. In the third type, speech is fluent and grammatically well formed, but the content of what the children say has an odd quality and the way in which they use language in social interactions is unusual. Initially termed 'semantic-pragmatic syndrome' (Rapin and Allen, 1983), 'semantic-pragmatic disorder' (Bishop and Rosenbloom, 1987) or 'conversational disability' (Conti-Ramsden and Gunn, 1986), this is now commonly referred to simply as pragmatic disorder (Bishop, 2000). It was apparent from the earliest accounts that children with this form of specific language impairment often display social and behavioural abnormalities similar to those seen in autism and Asperger's syndrome.

Bishop and Adams (1989; see also Bishop, 1997) attempted to identify what it was that caused the speech of children with pragmatic disorder to appear odd. They gathered conversational data from fourteen such children aged eight to twelve by showing them photographs, for example, of a doctor examining a sick boy and a girl having a birthday party, and asking them to talk about their own similar experiences. The conversations were transcribed and rated for indications of 'inappropriacy', odd or unexpected utterances where the smooth flow of conversation broke down.

One such characteristic was a failure, similar to that described above in autistic patients, to understand the implied meaning of an utterance, For example:

Would you say the boy looked ill?
The boy looked ill.

However, this was uncommon, and the same phenomenon was also seen in a control group of younger normal children. Other types of inappropriate response, however, were seldom seen in normally developing children of any age. One of these was a tendency to provide the listener with too little or too much information. High scores on both indices often co-existed in the same child. The children with pragmatic disorder also had markedly higher ratings than children with other forms of specific language impairment on unusual or socially inappropriate content or style, which included stereotyped and formulaic language, inappropriate questioning and socially inappropriate remarks. Some of the children also showed topic shifts. However, this characteristically consisted of steering any and all conversations round to their own circumscribed interests.

Although the children were often described as verbose, they did not produce an unusually high rate of utterances per turn. The impression of wordiness seemed to reflect the unusual content of their utterances, in which they produced unnecessary repetitions, asserted or denied what was already known, or gave precise and over-elaborate information.

From Rumsey et al.'s study the main speech and thought abnormalities in high functioning adult autistic patients, and so presumably also those with Asperger's syndrome, are poverty of speech and poverty of content of speech. Circumstantiality and stiltedness did not feature in Rumsey's study, but abnormalities which probably correspond to these clinical terms have been found in the children with pragmatic disorder studied by Bishop and Adams. The relationship between these two disorders is close, to the extent that it is controversial whether pragmatic speech disorder ever occurs outside children without other evidence of autism or Asperger's syndrome, although current evidence favours a degree of dissociation (Bishop, 2000). One consequence of this closeness has been that it has become universally accepted that many if not all of the language difficulties of autistic and Asperger patients can be understood as an impairment in pragmatics (see Chapter 5).

Thought disorder in normal individuals

Authors writing about thought disorder invariably make the point, usually without much elaboration, that something akin to thought disorder can be sometimes seen as a normal phenomenon. One variation on this theme is that normal people may become thought-disordered when they are tired or under stress. Another is that certain people without any diagnosable mental illness habitually speak fluent nonsense. Finally, as alluded to at the beginning of the chapter, something at least superficially similar to thought disorder is apparent in the works of certain poets and writers, where its obscurity is presumed to be at least to some extent the result of conscious creative effort.

The idea that almost anyone can become thought-disordered under the right conditions has been widely perpetuated but poorly documented. One of the very few, but also one of the neatest, illustrations of this occurrence was provided by Schwartz (1982), in the form of the following transcript of a normal subject talking while probably tired and definitely under more than a little stress. Schwartz considered it to be repetitive, loose and difficult to follow, although lacking the bizarre quality of schizophrenic loose associations. Several of his clinical psychologist colleagues nevertheless rated it as 'moderately schizophrenic'.

Well I wonder if that part of it can't be – I wonder if that doesn't – let me put it frankly; I wonder if that doesn't have to be continued? Let me put it this way: let us suppose you get the million bucks, and you get the proper way to handle it. You could hold that side?

In fact, the individual concerned had every reason to be tired and under stress, as he was Richard Nixon talking to his aides about the Watergate scandal which was shortly to bring down his presidency and put several of them in jail.

To be less than coherent when tired, anxious, etc., is one thing; to fail to speak coherently on a routine basis is another. Several authors have implied that such individuals exist, but actual examples are even harder to track down than those of thought disorder under conditions of stress. One of the present authors has encountered the phenomenon perhaps twice in twenty-five years. The more striking case was the husband of a patient who had been admitted to hospital with depression. He worked as a tailor and had no history of any psychiatric or neurological disorder. When interviewed about his wife's illness he launched into waves of bizarre, high-sounding and completely incomprehensible speech which appeared (at least to the author at a time when he was not very experienced) indistinguishable from thought disorder as seen in schizophrenia. His wife did not seem to feel that his speech was unusual.

It would of course be too much to expect that anyone would have rated such non-psychiatrically ill, thought-disordered individuals using the TLC scale, but surprisingly a study with something approximating to this design has been carried out. Having become interested in the largely uninvestigated phenomenon of eccentricity, Weeks and co-workers (Weeks and Ward, 1988; Weeks and James, 1995) attempted to recruit a sample of such individuals by placing cards in libraries, pubs, supermarkets, universities and so on. This read: 'Eccentric? If you feel that you might be, contact Dr David Weeks at the Royal Edinburgh Hospital' and gave a telephone number. This led to a certain amount of press interest, and ultimately the study received national and then international media coverage. They were able to recruit a sample of 789 potential eccentrics by this means, and eventually the number grew to more than a thousand. As Weeks and James (1995) described them:

The subjects ranged across the entire social spectrum, including a deputy chairman of a large industrial firm, a senior judge, a puppeteer, a chiropractor and an unemployed poet. There were several self-made millionaires and a few cave-dwelling hermits. There were housewives and sorceresses, university professors and factory workers, computer scientists and established artists and writers.

All the subjects were interviewed using the Present State Examination, supplemented by open-ended questioning aimed at drawing out as complete answers as possible. Tape recordings of the interviews were then rated using the TLC scale. Two thirds of the sample showed no abnormality of thought form, but in the remainder speech had a distinctly odd ring, although it was usually decipherable. Pressure of speech, circumstantiality and tangentiality were the most frequently rated abnormalities and reflected a characteristic long-windedness and flowery use of language. Self-reference was also present in 28%, much higher than the rates found in schizophrenia and mania by Andreasen (1979c); even in informal conversations about neutral topics, eccentrics tended to refer the conversation back to themselves repeatedly. Two items, derailment and loss of goal, were rated less frequently than in Andreasen's normal subjects. This was considered to reflect the eccentrics' single-mindedness about their various hobbyhorses, which occasionally extended to their following the interviewer out of the room to continue discussing them. Or as Weeks and James (1995) put it 'eccentrics are mildly deficient in normal digressiveness'.

The speech of a few of the subjects was frankly incoherent. Two examples are shown in Box 3.5, where stiltedness, poverty of content, derailment and idiosyncratic use of words is apparent, plus, in the first extract, a single possible instance of clanging (peace . . . peas). These subjects were not psychotic at the time of examination, and neither had any history of psychiatric illness. In fact formal psychiatric illness was uncommon in the sample as a whole: one subject was schizophrenic, one had a history of bipolar disorder, a few had had previous episodes of depression, and there were a number with alcohol-related problems.

Box 3.5 Thought disorder in eccentric but not mentally ill individuals

(From Weeks and Ward, 1988, reproduced with permission)

Your trained mind could tolerate my ineffectuality of knowledge . . . You may gladly have the bones of my lifetime journey . . . Biology made me an ineffectual creature-spirit, brooding over chaos. I longed to be an artist. My sensitivity turned into 100 per cent pacifism, befitting my physical ummanliness, deemed cowardice. So be it . . . I did not make myself . . . My errors may have compounded my naivete lack of worldly wise. To add fear to fearfulness is cruelty. Thought has been a permanent friend . . . and enemy . . . to try and reason with lifelong regret of ignorance of life and how it is lived. *Why* is the one word always with me.

Inflationally richer in ertz [ʔersatz] money, and to have learned what little impact the born introverted mind has on society, the eccentric can be consoled of their bijou part through life, which the gregarious have made less secure than the simplicity of my childhood. No earth could he more wonderful, no altruism, so trampled by the sheer forces opposing peace . . . and harmony . . . which the populist mind chooses as its rights. Why I even got into the pod of civilization's green peas, ancestry alone knows.

(Brendan, age sixty-six)

[In response to the question, Are you a collector?] Yes. I do . . . the collection comes down to this . . . If someone says to me I have a rhyme for your CB broadcast . . . my first answer would be . . . did you? . . . Or the question would be . . . did you do it yourself? Now I am interested if he or she did it themselves . . . It doesn't matter what it sounds like, what is of interest to me is what it sounds like, but it is more important that they did it themselves. If it is something, say Wordsworth . . . then I am sorry, I am not interested. I am only interested in the immediate . . . what you or yours experience. If I want Wordsworth then I suppose I would go and get him and explain it to myself one way or another, but I don't want that, but I do want this one. That is the difference . . . I collect that . . . I don't collect Wordsworth, but I do collect the aspiring or the clever.

I will take anything – virtually the most prosaic thing, and I can kick it into a story, for instance, verses really to me are little stories, it just so happens that I put

> them into verse, maybe one verse. If so then these are the most difficult, because you have to get a beginning, a middle and an end, all in one verse – if you have got more – I take any subject like that. (Leo, age forty-five)

Andreasen's (1979a,c) statement that thought disorder may occur in highly creative individuals such as writers was not an idle remark. For one thing, it was informed by her own study described above (Andreasen *et al.*, 1974), which demonstrated that professionals working with psychiatric patients could not reliably distinguish schizophrenic thought disorder from certain well-regarded literary productions. For another, prior to becoming a psychiatrist, Andreasen had been a lecturer in English Literature.[8]

Several authors, such as Critchley (1964), Forrest (1965) and Reed (1970), have pondered the link between thought-disordered schizophrenic speech and creative writing, generally to the effect that they may draw on the same well-springs, but that, while the former is spontaneous, constant revision is necessary to achieve the latter. Writers cited in the service of these arguments have included Dylan Thomas, Gertrude Stein, E. E. Cummings and even Shakespeare. However, the colossus in this particular field has always been James Joyce. His two great novels, *Ulysses* and *Finnegans Wake*, are to say the least difficult to follow, in contrast to his relatively conventional earlier work. *Ulysses* was well received when it was published, sold well and went on to make Joyce the most important figure in twentieth-century literature. *Finnegans Wake*, in contrast, was published to generally poor reviews and even Joyce's literary friends seemed to find it largely incomprehensible. Arnold (1969) described the way in which *Ulysses* was written as follows:

> On the average, Joyce wrote about half a page (of the final version) per day. The time-consuming things were collecting information, organizing the material, thinking out the symbolisms and parallelisms, and revising what had already been written in the light of new themes or techniques introduced in later episodes. The book grew in size by a third while in proof. *Ulysses* is a repository of all the things Joyce knew – what he had learned in school, what he had read, what he had been told by others, what he himself had experienced.

Joyce's technique for writing *Finnegans Wake*, which took sixteen years to complete, was similar but went further. Each draft became more and more obscure as, once again in the words of Arnold (1969), 'he revised, made changes, obscured meanings, twisted words, and wrote new parts'. The spelling of many words was changed over successive drafts to make them more unconventional, or to engage in

---

[8] On occasion Andreasen has been able to put her literary knowledge to good use. For example, when a psychiatrist giving a talk on the topic of depression in schizophrenia wondered whether, as Voltaire put it, chronic schizophrenics, like the mass of men, live lives of quiet desperation, she called out in a shocked voice from the front row, 'It was Thoreau!'

> **Box 3.6** The opening paragraphs of Finnegans Wake and Joyce's key to some of it
>
> (From Arnold, 1969)
>
> riverrun, past Eve and Adam's, from swerve of shore to bend of bay, brings us by a commodius vicus of recirculation back to Howth Castle and Environs.
>
>   Sir Tristram, violer d'amores, fr'over the short sea, had passencore rearrived from North 'Armorica on this side the scraggy isthmus of Europe Minor to wielderfight his penisolate war: nor had topsawyer's rocks by the stream Oconee exaggerated themselse to Laurens County's gorgios while they went doublin their mumper all the time: nor avoice from afire bellowsed mishe mishe to tauftauf thuartpeatrick:
>
> passencore = pas encore and ricorsi storici of Vico North Armorica = Brittany
> wielderfight = wielderfecten = refight
> Dublin, Laurens Co, Georgia, founded by a Dubliner, Peter Sawyer, on the river Oconee. Its motto: Doubling all the time
> Mishe = I am (Irish) i.e. Christian tauf = to baptize (German)
> thuartpeatrick = Thou art Peter and upon this rock etc.
>
> (The first half of the first sentence is believed to be the unfinished last sentence of the book.)

puns and word play, to make them refer to other happenings in the book, or to permit several meanings to be discovered in them – for example incest was always spelled as insect; penisolate embodied penis, Isolde, pen, peninsula war, etc. Some words were written back to front, e.g, rabworc for crowbar.

    Joyce sent an early version of a passage which became the opening paragraph of *Finnegans Wake* to a friend, helpfully adding a key which was itself almost completely opaque. This is reproduced in Box 3.6.

    Although he would probably qualify for a diagnosis of alcoholism, as would his father, Joyce did not suffer from anything recognisable as mental illness at any point in his life. He was arrogant and had a high opinion of his literary prowess even before he wrote his first novel, and throughout his life he had serious quarrels with people, often those who had helped him in significant ways. It has been stated that he complained of hearing voices after prolonged drinking bouts, but the source for this claim is difficult to track down, and no other symptoms or behaviours suggestive of psychosis have ever been recorded. The letters he wrote up to the time of his death were all completely lucid. A series of conversations with a friend, reconstructed from notes taken at the time (Power, 1974), also appear to have been perfectly understandable from the time he wrote *Ulysses* until shortly before his death.

So, Joyce's later writings, it seems, were the result of a deliberate, even painstaking process of successive revision, which was used to brilliant effect in *Ulysses*, but was perhaps taken too far in *Finnegans Wake*; any resemblance to thought disorder is purely coincidental. This reassuring conclusion is thrown into a certain amount of disarray by the fact that his daughter, Lucia, suffered from a mental illness which was in all probability schizophrenia. As described in Ellman's (1959) comprehensive biography of Joyce, she showed increasingly odd and disturbed behaviour from around the age of twenty-two, and was first hospitalised at the age of twenty-four. She failed to make a complete recovery, and afterwards was outspoken and abrasive with friends and family. She spent further time in sanatoriums and clinics, where she was at times apathetic and dreamy and at other times prone to violence or sudden impulsive acts. She became chronically hospitalised at the age of thirty-six and spent the rest of her life in institutional care. A friend of the family (Lidderdale, 1983), who kept in contact with her until she died, described her as remaining very disturbed until new drugs enabled her to lead a more or less normal life within the shelter of the hospital. She was given a number of different diagnoses in the early years of her illness, and a recent biographer (Shloss, 2003) has argued that she did not suffer from mental illness in the customary meaning of the term. Nevertheless, the Irish schizophrenia support organisation is named after her.

It would be an intriguing and even Joycean note to end on to be able to state that Lucia Joyce showed thought disorder. Certainly, it has been said that in the first few years of her illness she showed breaks in her conversation and swift jumps of thought which baffled people, but which Joyce himself showed a remarkable capacity to follow (Ellman, 1959). Jung, who briefly treated her, also referred to her use of neologisms and portmanteau words (Ellman, 1959; Shloss, 2003). But the reality is that her symptoms have never been described in detail, and her medical records are not available for scrutiny. Neither the letters which survive from the early years of her illness (many were destroyed) nor the few longer pieces she wrote when she was older show anything more than a mild vagueness and disjointedness.

4

Thought disorder as a form of dysphasia

As a highly researched symptom of schizophrenia, theories of thought disorder have abounded in the past and continue in steady supply to the present day. These have run the familiar psychiatric gamut from the psychodynamic – for instance that schizophrenic patients are speaking in metaphors to describe their strange inner world, or that they are expressing a pattern of deviant communication learnt from their parents – to the biological, which in one way or another try to explain thought disorder in terms of a disturbance of function in one or more brain regions. As the current mainstream view is that schizophrenia is a biological disease, these latter approaches are now the dominant ones, and the most important of them are discussed in the next three chapters. But of all the approaches, easily the most unpopular has been the proposal that thought disorder is a disorder of language, specifically of language in its most basic sense, the kind of language disturbance which, when it occurs in neurological patients, is called dysphasia.

Although a number of names have subsequently become attached to it, the idea that thought disorder could be a form of dysphasia can be traced to the work of a single individual, who was its most tenacious adherent over the years and often a target of vilification for expressing it. This was Kleist.

The fons et origio

Kleist (see Box 4.1) was a psychiatrist who worked in Germany from the beginning of the twentieth century, a country where there was, and still is, less of a division between psychiatry and neurology than in Britain and America. His views on thought disorder are contained in three papers (Kleist, 1914, 1930, 1960), the first of which gave by far the most detailed account. Beginning with the assertion that speech disorders were not confined to illnesses with a recognisable brain localisa-tion, 'but occur also in brain disorders of a more general kind, that is in mental illnesses', Kleist (1914) went on to state that patients with schizophrenia afforded the best material for the study of these. In his experience, while comprehension of speech was not disturbed in the disorder, it was possible to identify abnormalities of speech expression similar to those seen in frontal motor aphasia (i.e. Broca's aphasia) and paraphasias similar to those seen in temporal lobe aphasia (i.e. Wernicke's aphasia).

Box 4.1 Who was Kleist?

(From Berrios, personal communication)

Karl Kleist (1879–1960) trained under Wernicke, who was a major influence on his views, and also worked briefly with Kraepelin. In the first world war he was the director of a neurological team caring for patients with head injuries due to missile wounds. He later became professor of neurology and psychiatry in Frankfurt and then Leipzig.

Despite the fact that most of his published work was on psychiatric topics, he made respected contributions to neurology. He coined or at least popularised the terms agrammatism and paragrammatism which are in routine use today to describe features of dysphasia. He also gave an early description of conduction aphasia. His observations on the frontal lobe syndrome are regularly cited. He also gave one of the original descriptions of constructional apraxia.

Kleist fundamentally disagreed with the simple Kraepelinian division of psychosis into schizophrenia and manic-depressive psychosis, and followed the rival approach of Wernicke, who believed that there were multiple discrete types of schizophrenia, that the concept of manic-depressive psychosis was too broad, and that there were forms of psychosis intermediate between the two. After Wernicke's untimely death, Kleist became the main proponent of this school of thought, and the tradition has in turn been kept alive by Leonhard. Although the whole Wernicke–Kleist–Leonhard classification has not stood the test of time, it has led to some significant advances, notably the distinction between unipolar and bipolar affective disorder, and the concept of cycloid psychosis, which is now included in ICD-10 as acute polymorphic psychotic disorder.

Kleist believed that the symptoms of psychosis were essentially similar to those produced by focal brain lesions, and could ultimately be understood as dysfunction of these regions. Because of this he was attacked by gestalt-influenced German psychiatrists in the 1920s. It did not help that he steadfastly refused to accept, or even acknowledge, the work of Freud. His argument that thought disorder was a form of aphasia grew out of this.

In a paper entitled 'Schizophrenic symptoms and cerebral pathology', published in the last year of his life, Kleist summarised his views on the brain regions implicated in schizophrenia. Leaving aside the brain stem, which he believed was related to certain delusional states, the brain areas he identified are for the most part those which now preoccupy schizophrenia research – the frontal lobes, the temporal lobes, the cingulate gyrus and the basal ganglia.

Motor speech disorders tended to be seen in catatonic patients, particularly those with his subtype of 'drive poor' catatonia, and took the form of difficulty pronouncing sounds, stumbling over syllables and repetitions. Such patients could also show agrammatism, the basic feature of which was the simplification and coarsening of word sequences. Kleist's description was similar in all respects to Broca's aphasia:

Complicated sentence constructions (subjugation of clauses) are impossible. Sufferers utter only small primitive sentences if any at all. Less necessary words, especially pronouns and particles, are reduced or eliminated altogether. In this sense agrammatism is similar to impoverishment of vocabulary. Conjugation, too, which is necessary for expressing different times and modi, declines. Word changes inherent in conjugation, declination and comparison more or less disappear. In severe cases only nouns and adjectives in the nominative and verbs in the infinitive and participle remain. These are joined in a crude sequence as children do when they change from single to multiple word expression.

In contrast, other patients, particularly those with paranoid or hebephrenic schizophrenia, showed a disorder marked by many paraphasias. In these cases it was extraordinary that there was no comprehension deficit ('word deafness') similar to that seen in Wernicke's aphasia. Some of these patients had difficulty finding words ('word amnesias'), but this played a minor role in comparison to its frequent occurrence in aphasia. Rather more frequently, the same words were used over and over again, for example one patient used the word 'build' for any kind of useful activity, and 'run' in the sense of 'reach' and 'be adequate', as in 'the branches of the tree are running far' or 'the coffee never runs', i.e. is never enough.

In addition, Kleist (1914) considered that schizophrenic patients showed other disorders which in his view were aphasic in nature, but were not seen in neurological patients. One of these was a disorder of word formation, where compounds and derivatives were formed from a small set of words or word fragments. A patient referred to a clock as a 'time container', a brush as a 'pluck container', a jug as a 'water container'; when asked what a law court was, she said it was a 'people container'. Often the words used were not static in meaning: the same patient described the fins of a fish as 'swimming wings', and a silhouette as 'fantasy dolls', 'night images' and 'night dolls'. A candle was described as a 'night illuminating object', a military insignia as 'service quality defined rank decoration'. Some of these disorders of word construction would be recognised today as circumlocutions; others as word approximations.

Also in this category was what Kleist called paragrammatism. Whereas agrammatism was mainly characterised by omission of auxiliary words, word inflections, prefixes and suffixes, in paragrammatism there was an incorrect use of these elements:

the ability to form word sequences is not lost, but phrases and sentences are often chosen incorrectly, get mixed up and contaminate one another. Started phrases and sentences are often not completed and so form anacolutha. Linguistic expression is not simplified but, combined with an overproduction of word sequences, exaggerated to produce confusing and monstrous language.

In 1930, based on his experience of caring for soldiers with head injuries in the First World War, Kleist went further, stating that 'patients with brain disease and war wounds in the left temporal lobe also demonstrated the same gross speech disorders – paraphasias and word amnesias, but also the same fine defects – the characteristic word errors, formation of new words and the strange formation of sentences – that one sees in schizophrenics.' By this time one of his colleagues had succeeded in showing that the comprehension of speech was also disturbed in schizophrenic patients, and Kleist believed that this demonstrated beyond doubt the sensory aphasic nature of some of their disorders of speech.[1]

At the same time he qualified this conclusion by stating: 'I have never believed that all the disordered speech in schizophrenics originates from an aphasia-like disturbance, only that such a disorder does exist in some patients.' Some of the additional disorders of thought were, in Kleist's view, also explicable in organic terms. One of these was alogia, a failure in the thinking process, which he believed was similar to symptoms seen in patients with brain damage affecting the left side of the brain, the frontal lobes or the brainstem. This was characterised by poverty and lack of productivity of thought. Such patients were incapable of producing coherent thoughts from single ideas or perceptions, and could not draw conclusions or point out similarities and differences among a range of facts. The other was paralogia, a breakdown in the conceptual processes underlying speech. Kleist defined this even less clearly than alogia but seemed to be describing a failure of the ability to make connections between concepts, which led them to be replaced by loosely connected ideas or to emerge in incomplete or fragmentary fashion.

In 1960, uncompromising to the end, and in the light of more neuropathological knowledge from the Second World War and the increasing number of road accidents, Kleist made an attempt to consider all schizophrenic symptoms from a neurological standpoint. With respect to the speech confused subtype of schizophrenia (see Chapter 2) he stated that one was 'dealing with *sensory aphasic impairments* similar to those found in focal brain lesions of the *left temporal lobe*' (italics in original). His only concession to orthodoxy was the acknowledgment that an additional 'higher-level' impairment seemed to be involved, which affected the formation of sentences and the abstract meaning of speech.

---

[1] All known forms of fluent aphasia are characterised not only by a disorder of expressed speech but also by impaired comprehension of speech, hence the importance Kleist attached to documenting this.

Patients with other subtypes of schizophrenia could show principally incoherence of thought rather than speech, but even in these cases paraphasias and paragrammatism were interspersed among the mental jumps.

Kleist's views on thought disorder came, even within his own lifetime, to be regarded as only of historical interest. In psychiatric and psychological circles he was mostly ignored. Neurologists cited his work more frequently, but only to demolish it, usually by appeal to their own clinical authority. Thus Critchley (1964) observed that 'resemblances there may be at times between the diction or writings of a schizophrenic and those of an aphasiac, but they must not be overstressed, and analogy must not be promoted to the level of a hypothesis', before going on to brand Kleist as a deviationist, a heretic and, more obscurely, a materialist. Another critic of Kleist's (Benson, 1973) noted that in his experience every case presented to him as a schizophrenic with word-salad ultimately proved to have fluent dysphasia caused by organic brain disease.

Enter Chaika

This complacent consensus persisted until it was shattered by a linguist, Chaika (1974), in a paper entitled 'A linguist looks at "schizophrenic" language'. She carried out a linguistic analysis on speech from a thirty-seven-year-old chronically hospitalised woman who had been repeatedly diagnosed as schizophrenic and had no evidence of neurological disease. The patient spoke in what was virtually a series of monologues, without pausing long enough to allow the listener to easily interrupt, although when asked a question she would answer. For example, as she entered the room, spied a packet of cigarettes, and picked it up, she said the following:

Good mornin' everybody! (lower pitch, doubtfully) I don't know what that is. (laughs). The(re) sawendon saw turch faw jueri. (Loudly, very surprised) Oh! it's that thorazine. I forgot I had it. That's Lulubelle. This one's Jean. J-E-A-N. I'll write that down. Speeds up the metabolism. Makes your life shorter. Makes your heart bong. Tranquillizes you if you've got the metabolism I have. I have distemper just like cats do, 'cause that's what we all are, felines. (Pause) Siamese cat balls. They stand out. I had a cat, a manx, still around somewhere. You'll know him when you see him. His name is GI Joe; he's black and white. I had a little goldfish too, like a clown. (Pause, drop to low pitch, as in an aside) Happy Halloween down. (Pause, higher pitch) dudn He still had fooch with teykrimez I'll be willing to betcha. Nobody takes my word for what I wanna do. Not even God. I believe I'll try anyhow. (declaiming) I believe in the spirit of the mountains. Right now I'm thinking Pike's Peak for a rehaul of the Korean thing. This time I'll marry E– P–, or 'bout H– G–? Or Frank Sinatra, he's already set.

Chaika began her analysis by redescribing several of the phenomena of thought disorder. She pointed out that the propositional content of individual sentences was usually understandable, but it was not subordinated to any subject matter. It also seemed probable that any of the semantic features of a word could determine the subsequent topic of discourse. Thus, discussing the tranquillising effect of thorazine perhaps made the patient think of temper, and then perhaps distemper. Distemper reminded her of cats, which reminded her of a kind of cat ball, which reminded her of her own pet cat, which reminded her of her goldfish. The phrase 'takes my word' seemed to trigger use of the word 'believe', which prompted her to use it in another meaning of having faith. This also extended to the phonetic features of words, as in 'Happy Halloween down', which rhymed with the preceding sentence, 'I had a little goldfish like a clown', as well as being possibly semantically associated.

Over and above this, Chaika described abnormalities which were more reminiscent of dysphasia. One of these was the patient's use of neologisms and what she called gibberish words. In each case these were uttered as if they were meaningful words, with no pause or stress before, during or after them. The words conformed to the phonological rules of English and the patient's dialect. In fact the words were so consistent with the stress and phonemic rules of English that, as Chaika put it, 'on first hearing, one thinks the patient has actually made utterances of the language which one has failed to catch'. Generally, the patient showed little disturbance in her syntax. However, in another segment of speech she did make one incontrovertible syntactic error, using the article 'a' instead of 'the':

In *a* month I've been upstairs, they've been taking my brains out a piece at a time or all together.

Finally, Chaika noted in passing an apparent lack of use of the discourse markers in connected speech necessary to show connections and orient listeners to her topic. This was to form the focus of considerable further research, which is discussed in the next chapter.

Chaika argued that these abnormalities were genuinely linguistic in nature and were indicative of a disturbance in those areas of the brain concerned with language. However, she was ambivalent about identifying thought disorder as a form of aphasia. Early in the paper she stated that the linguistic abnormalities discoverable in schizophrenic speech differed from other kinds of linguistic deviance, such as that occurring in poetry or in aphasia; later, however, she argued that if a schizophrenic patient's use of abnormal language was outside conscious control, then he or she 'is suffering from some sort of intermittent aphasia'.

Even with these qualifications and reservations, Chaika's (1974) study was enough to launch a debate among linguists. Fromkin (1975) attacked her conclusion that the abnormalities she described reflected a breakdown in language. Her argument was essentially that normal individuals often coin neologisms, for example in the use of slang; that they occasionally produce gibberish words when they make slips of the tongue; and that there is nothing very remarkable about syntactic errors, which were anyway infrequent in Chaika's patient. Lecours and Vanier-Clément (1976) carried out a series of case studies of their own. They concluded that, on the one hand, some of the paraphasias and neologisms which could be observed both in schizophrenia and certain forms of jargon aphasia, were linguistically indistinguishable from each other. On the other hand, in their view, many schizophrenic neologisms were quite different in nature from dysphasic neologisms, being based on unusual word choice rather than paraphasic substitution. They also argued that the production of sentences whose verbal components were based either on phonological or semantic associations outside the topic of conversation was not a feature of dysphasia. Herbert and Waltensperger (1980) weighed in with a schizophrenic patient who showed some but not all of the linguistic aberrations described by Chaika, but who showed much more marked grammatical abnormality: 'I'm was railroad'; 'Dr– turned in I'm understand the truth is the books to you'; '[they] give me cholera without me know'. Hoffman and Sledge (1984) also described a patient in whom they considered paragrammatisms to be prominent. Discussing the consequences of being left back a grade in school he said: 'That's why, you know, the fact that I did there was no stigmatism attached to that clearly explained in the record why you were put back, you know, um, or put-and/or put ahead, both.'

Confirmation of the dysphasia hypothesis?

Chaika (1974), if not exactly careful with her words, stopped short of claiming that thought disorder was a form of dysphasia. But now that the subject had been broached, some investigators were prepared to go further. Faber et al. (1983)[2] recorded interviews with fourteen thought-disordered schizophrenic patients, and thirteen patients with dysphasia (which was fluent in eleven cases and non-fluent in the remaining two). They then made transcripts of the interviews, from which all potentially identifying information, such as references to age, psychiatric or neurological symptoms and treatment, was removed, and presented them under blind conditions to two psychiatrists, two neurologists and a speech and language pathologist. None of these classified all the transcripts correctly. Neither of the neurologists scored significantly above chance (both were correct in 18/27 cases). The psychiatrists performed somewhat better (correct in 20/27 and 22/27 cases). The speech pathologist did best of all (correct in 25/27 cases), but even she was not completely successful. The speech pathologist's success was based on

---

[2] The authors of this study included Taylor and Abrams, two of American psychiatry's most dedicated controversialists.

observations that the schizophrenic patients were fluent, showed adequate auditory comprehension of questions and used multisyllabic words, whereas the aphasic patients showed comprehension deficits, word finding problems, impaired naming and used a reduced number of nouns. But even so the distinction was not always easy, as two examples from Faber *et al.*'s study show. The first is from an aphasic patient:

Dr. How are those men sick?
Pt. I don't know. A lot of times I went out there and told them, shook them up after I come over here, was here and having a little program here about in certain programs here and, ah, when I'd leave and go over to get the bus to go home, to get home downtown where I live at, I'd walk out the door out there and they'd be two or three stretched out there and in the grass out there and I would go out there and shake them up by the arm and everything, and that little nurse came out by the door and seen me stretching them out. She said: 'Mr–, don't touch them doofers no more.'

And the second is from a schizophrenic patient:

Dr. I don't follow you.
Pt. You don't follow the hemlock trees? I'm trying not to dig into the thing but ah, see, Johnson Anderson died before time. He could have died a little after time, Johnson Anderson the vault, let's see. I think it's see and, ah, you know, the middle of the mackers in the cemetery.

The speech pathologist also categorised the specific types of linguistic and thought abnormality she found in each transcript under blind conditions. These findings are shown in Table 4.1, from which it can be seen that the schizophrenic patients were commonly considered to show paraphasias and the dysphasic patients were almost as frequently rated as showing poverty of content of speech.

Later, the same group (Landre *et al.*, 1992) administered a selection of standard screening tests for dysphasia to ten thought-disordered schizophrenic patients and ten patients with fluent aphasia. One was a test of comprehension of syntax, the Modified Token Test (DeRenzi and Faglioni, 1978), in which the subject has to follow instructions concerning shapes of different colour and size, which are increasingly grammatically complex (e.g. *Touch a circle. Instead of the white square, touch the yellow circle*). Another was the repetition of words and phrases subtests from the Boston Diagnostic Aphasia Examination (BDAE) (Goodglass and Kaplan, 1983/1994). The third was the Boston Naming Test from the same battery, in which the subjects have to name sixty words of increasing difficulty. Although, as can be seen from Figure 4.1, more of the aphasic patients showed severely impaired levels of performance, the two groups did not differ significantly on any of the tests. Landre *et al.* also noted that the schizophrenic patients' errors on the Boston Naming Test frequently included paraphasic or circumlocutory responses, such as 'atlas' for globe, 'stints' for stilts, and 'something you knock on' for door knocker.

Table 4.1 Language abnormalities rated blindly in dysphasic patients and schizophrenic patients with formal thought disorder

(From Faber *et al.*, *American Journal of Psychiatry*, **140**, 1348–1351, 1983. Copyright 1983, the American Psychiatric Association, http://ajp.psychiatryonline.org. Reprinted by permission.)

	Dysphasic patients ($n = 13$)	Schizophrenic patients ($n = 14$)	P value
Paraphasias	8	9	NS
Agrammatism	2	0	NS
Impaired comprehension of speech	5	0	0.04
Anomia/word finding problems	7	0	0.01
Pronoun word problems	4	0	NS
Circumlocutions	1	0	NS
Neologisms	1	3	NS
Word approximations/idiosyncratic use of words	0	8	0.01
Perseveration	1	4	NS
Incoherence	3	10	NS
Derailment/tangentiality	2	11	0.05
Poverty of content	8	1	0.04
Illogicality	1	5	NS
Clanging	0	3	NS

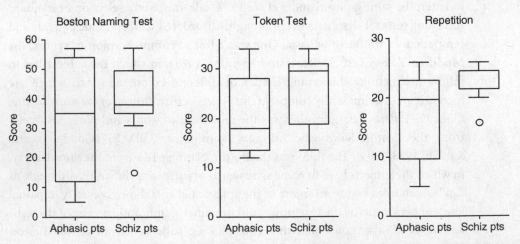

Figure 4.1   Distribution of scores on three aphasia tests for ten schizophrenic and ten aphasic patients (from Landre *et al.*, 1992, reproduced with permission)

The confounding factor of general intellectual impairment

Landre *et al.*'s (1992) study had a weakness, in that they failed to include a comparison group of non-thought-disordered schizophrenic patients. It might seem unlikely that language test performance would be affected in patients without any clinical disturbance of speech, but Faber and Reichstein (1981) had found clear indications that this was in fact the case in an earlier similar study: while a group of thought-disordered patients performed significantly more poorly than normal controls on six out of ten language tests, their performance was not significantly worse than that of a group of non-thought-disordered patients on seven of the tests.

Why should patients without thought disorder also perform poorly on language tests? The answer is simply that, as a group, patients with schizophrenia show some degree of general intellectual impairment. This in itself will cause poor performance on language tests, just as it would on memory, frontal, visual and any other specific neuropsychological test. In short, the impairment these two studies found might be nothing to do with the presence of thought disorder, but merely a reflection of the general tendency to poor cognitive test performance, which would show itself on any test.

To be fair, there was no more than a dim appreciation of general intellectual impairment in schizophrenia at the time Faber and Reichstein (1981) carried out their study, and ten years later Landre *et al.* (1992) did acknowledge that the language impairment they found might be part of a more generalised cognitive deficit. What is more difficult to excuse is the way psychiatry resolutely ignored the whole issue of cognitive impairment in schizophrenia until comparatively recently. The finding that patients with schizophrenia performed poorly on virtually any cognitive task was first documented in the 1930s (e.g. Chapman and Chapman, 1973) and was reinforced by a wave of studies using IQ tests in the 1940s (e.g. Payne, 1960), and then again by studies employing neuropsychological test batteries in the 1960s and 1970s (e.g. Heaton *et al.*, 1978). Yet it remained a finding that dare not speak its name until the 1980 biological coup in American psychiatry, described in Chapter 1, removed some of the barriers to its acceptance.[3]

Since then, the neuropsychology of schizophrenia has become a large and actively researched topic. A summary of the current state of knowledge, which avoids most of the controversies in the area, would be as follows. There is a variable tendency to poor cognitive performance in schizophrenia, which is most simply understood as reflecting a degree of general intellectual impairment associated with the disorder.

---

[3] Even so, five years later when Cutting (1985) wanted to call a book he had written, *The Neuropsychology of Schizophrenia* his publishers insisted he change it to *The Psychology of Schizophrenia* on the grounds that there would be no market for a book with his preferred title.

This shows itself in a lowering of IQ, and as an apparent decline from estimated levels of IQ functioning before the onset of illness (Barber *et al.*, 1996). A minority of patients show more severe degrees of general intellectual impairment, which can be detected by relatively crude clinical measures of cognitive function, such as the ubiquitous Mini-Mental State Examination (MMSE) of Folstein *et al.* (1975). An even smaller minority are profoundly impaired and show what is to all intents and purposes dementia (Owens and Johnstone, 1980; Liddle and Crow, 1984; DeVries *et al.*, 2002). Evidence suggests that the impairment is not due to neuroleptic drug treatment (e.g. King, 1990; Mortimer, 1997), and it has been documented in drug-free and never-treated patients (Saykin *et al.*, 1992, 1994). Within the general pattern, long-term memory and executive function may be disproportionately impaired and visual perception and verbal short-term memory may be relatively spared (McKenna *et al.*, 2002; Goldberg and Gold, 1995); however, no areas of function are completely unaffected (Heinrichs and Zakzanis, 1998). Broadly speaking, schizophrenic cognitive impairment is a function of severity and chronicity of illness, although there are many patients with chronic, severe illness who do not show marked impairment, and conversely patients who are not severely symptomatic occasionally show quite marked deficits.

The range and severity of neuropsychological test impairment in schizophrenia can be illustrated, in a way that is particularly relevant to studies described later in this chapter, by means of the neuropsychological case study approach used by Shallice *et al.* (1991). They administered tests of general intellectual function plus a wide range of specific neuropsychological tests to five chronically hospitalised patients. As shown in Table 4.2, the patients showed varying degrees of general intellectual impairment: HE and HS were relatively intact, as measured by a lack of a marked discrepancy between estimated premorbid IQ[4] and current IQ, and performance which was in the normal range on a non-verbal IQ test, Raven's matrices. RS showed somewhat more evidence of general intellectual impairment. LE and GT showed a marked IQ decline and were grossly impaired on Raven's Matrices. HE and HS tended to pass most of the specific neuropsychological tests, whereas the remaining patients showed more failures, which increased with increasing degrees of general intellectual impairment. Nevertheless, even the intellectually preserved patients showed some failures on the specific tests; these were principally on tests of frontal or executive functioning, leading Shallice *et al.* to argue that this was the common denominator of schizophrenic cognitive impairment.

---

[4] Based on the National Adult Reading Test (NART) of Nelson (1982). This tests ability to pronounce words, such as *gaol*, *zealot* and *desmesne*, which do not follow normal rules of pronunciation. Being able to pronounce a word is a good indicator that its meaning is also known, even if this latter knowledge has been lost due to, say, dementia.

Table 4.2 The profile of neuropsychological impairment in five chronically hospitalised schizophrenic patients

(From Shallice *et al.*, 1991)

	HE	HS	RS	LE	GT
Age	44	66	55	44	38
Estimated premorbid IQ (NART)	122	111	110	104	94
Current IQ (WAIS)	108	104	100	76	69
Raven's progressive matrices	0	1	3	3	3
Visual/visuospatial function					
Figure-ground discrimination	0	0	0	3	0
Dot centring	0	0	0	0	3
Dot counting	0	0	0	0	0
Cube analysis	0	0	0	0	2
Unusual views	0	0	3	3	3
Usual views	0	0	3	3	3
Recognition from silhouettes	0	2	2	3	3
Figure copy	0	2	0	0	3
Language					
Graded naming test	0	0	0	1	3
Naming from description	1	0	3	3	3
Modified Token Test	0	0	3	3	3
Memory					
Digit span	0	0	0	1	1
Story recall (immediate)	3	0	3	1	3
Figure recall (immediate)	0	0	1	3	3
List learning	3	1	3	3	3
Paired associates	0	0	3	–	3
Recognition memory (words)	0	0	2	0	1
Recognition memory (faces)	0	0	0	1	3
Executive function					
Alternation task	0	0	3	0	3
Cognitive Estimates Test	3	0	3	3	3
Modified Wisconsin Card Sorting Test	3	0	3	1	1
Money's Road Map Test	0	3	3	3	3
Personal orientation test	0	0	3	3	3
Self-ordered pointing	0	3	3	3	3
Stroop: colour naming	2	3	0	3	3
Trail Making Test (B)	3	2	0	3	3

Table 4.2 (cont.)

	HE	HS	RS	LE	GT
Verbal fluency (FAS Test)	0	1	2	0	0
Weigl–Golstein–Scheerer sort	0	3	0	3	3
Total no. of tests failed	**5**	**4**	**13**	**15**	**21**

Notes: Not all the memory tests are shown, due to the large number of these. Scores 0–3 are impairment indexes derived from normative data. 0 = at or above 25th percentile; 1 = 10–25th percentile; 2 = 5–10th percentile; 3 = below 5th percentile, the usual criterion for failure.

More studies using aphasia test batteries

Two very similar studies (Blakey *et al.*, 1996; Rodriguez-Ferrera *et al.*, 2001) asked the question of whether impairment on linguistic tests in schizophrenia was a function of thought disorder or general intellectual impairment. They administered a range of standard aphasia tests, plus measures of general intellectual function, to groups of thirty and forty schizophrenic patients respectively. Thought disorder was rated using the TLC scale. In both studies performance on virtually all the language tests was significantly correlated with general intellectual measures like MMSE score and current IQ, but on the whole there was no relationship with thought disorder. Rodriguez-Ferrera *et al.* found that thought disorder did correlate significantly with performance on two language tests: an expressive test, picture description and a test of semantic comprehension, the Pyramids and Palm Trees Test (Howard and Patterson, 1992). There was also a correlation with a test of syntactic comprehension, the Test for Reception of Grammar, although this did not survive when the more exacting statistical technique of multiple regression was used rather than correlation.

Oh *et al.* (2002) attempted to disentangle the effects of thought disorder and intellectual impairment on linguistic test performance using the single case study approach of Shallice *et al.* (1991). Out of a population of approximately 200 chronic schizophrenic patients, they selected six who showed severe thought disorder; these all received global ratings of 4 or 5 on the TLC scale, and had all shown the symptom consistently for years. They also examined seven patients who received global ratings of 0 or 1 on the TLC scale. The two sets of patients were comparable in terms of age, and all were of at least average estimated premorbid IQ. As in Shallice *et al.*'s study, the patients spanned a wide range of current intellectual functioning, from intact – i.e. estimated premorbid/current IQ discrepancies of less than 15 points plus MMSE scores close to the maximum of 30 – to very impaired – i.e. estimated premorbid/current IQ discrepancies of over 40 points and MMSE scores just above the cutoff of 23/24 for mild dementia.

Both sets of patients were given a range of tests from the BDAE. The pattern of performance in the thought-disordered and non-thought-disordered patients is shown in Tables 4.3a and 4.3b. Test failures were scattered and relatively infrequent. The overall failure rate was not greatly different in the two groups – the thought-disordered patients failed twenty-one out of ninety tests (23.3%) and the non-thought-disordered patients failed twenty out of 105 (19.0%). As in the study of Shallice *et al.* (1991), test failures in both groups also tended to increase with increasing degrees of general intellectual impairment. Thus the intellectually well-preserved patients at the left of Tables 4.3a and 4.3b only failed one or two tests, whereas the most severely intellectually impaired patients at the extreme right failed six and nine tests respectively. This tendency appeared to apply to most of the tests used. One apparent exception was visual confrontation naming. Here, however, the high failure rate in both groups was due to slowness of responding in all cases rather than naming errors. Slowness of responding is a well-recognised aspect of schizophrenic cognitive performance, and so this finding is not surprising.

Table 4.3 Performance of schizophrenic patients with and without thought disorder on the Boston Diagnostic Aphasia Examination and the Boston Naming Test

(From Oh *et al.*, 2002)

(a) Thought-disordered patients

BDAE	HC	EP	RR	SO	MA	TC
Word discrimination (72)	66.2*	68	72	62*	66*	60*
Body part identification (20)	19	19	20	19	19	20
Commands (15)	15	15	14	8*	15	7*
Complex ideational material (12)	11	5*	5*	5*	9	2*
Automatized sequences (8)	8	8	7	8	7	7
Recitation (2)	2	2	0*	2	2	2
Rhythm (2)	1	1	2	1	1	1
Repetition of words (10)	10	10	10	10	10	10
Repetition of phrases:						
High frequency (8)	8	8	7	8	8	8
Low frequency (8)	8	8	6	6	4*	8
Word reading (30)	30	30	30	30	30	27[†]
Responsive naming (30)	29	30	30	24[†]	30	26[†]
Visual confrontation naming (114)	110[†]	98[†]	99[†]	95[†]	111[†]	108[†]
Oral sentence reading (10)	10	10	10	9	9	9
Reading sentences/paragraphs (10)	9	7	9	7	7	7
No. of tests failed	**2**	**2**	**3**	**5**	**3**	**6**
Boston Naming Test (60)	57	55	49	51	54	47

Table 4.3 (cont.)

(b) Non-thought-disordered patients

BDAE	RC	CN	SB	RW	JA	RA	JJ
Word discrimination (72)	71	70	72	72	72	70	66*
Body part identification (20)	19.5	18.5	20	20	20	20	15*
Commands (15)	15	15	13	14	15	12*	10*
Complex ideational material (12)	10	7*	7*	10	5*	8	1*
Automatized sequences (8)	8	7	8	8	8	6	8
Recitation (2)	2	2	2	2	2	2	2
Rhythm (2)	1	1	2	1	2	1	0*
Repetition of words (10)	10	10	10	10	10	9	8*
Repetition of phrases:							
High frequency (8)	8	8	8	8	8	7	6
Low frequency (8)	7	8	7	8	8	4*	3*
Word reading (30)	30	30	30	30	30	30	29[†]
Responsive naming (30)	30	30	27	30	27	30	29
Visual confrontation naming (114)	111[†]	113[†]	111[†]	110[†]	114	108[†]	111[†]
Oral sentence reading (10)	9	10	10	10	10	9	10
Reading sentences/paragraphs (10)	10	9	9	10	8	6*	7
No. of tests failed	**1**	**2**	**2**	**1**	**1**	**4**	**9**
Boston Naming Test (60)	52	53	–	59	53	39*	35*

Notes: Maximum scores in brackets.
*Test failed on basis of score below BDAE cutoff.
[†]Test failed on basis of slowness only.

The naming tests in the BDAE are very simple, but the battery also includes the more demanding Boston Naming Test. None of the thought-disordered patients failed this test. Two non-thought-disordered patients failed; these were RA and JJ, who showed the greatest degrees of general intellectual impairment in this group.

More studies of expressive speech

The studies of Blakey *et al.*, Rodriguez-Ferrera *et al.* and Oh *et al.* effectively destroy any case for a disorder of comprehension and naming in thought disorder. Impairment on these tests is a function of intellectual impairment – unsurprisingly, as it seems unlikely that the general tendency to poor cognitive test performance in schizophrenia could somehow spare the specific area of language – and is seen in thought-disordered and non-thought-disordered patients alike. It remains possible, however, that thought disorder is associated with a disorder of language expression. While this would be unprecedented for dysphasia, in fluent forms of which impaired comprehension and abnormal expression invariably go hand in hand, Kleist's (1914) original observations meant that schizophrenic speech was always likely to be an exception to this rule.

Morice and Ingram (1982) carried out a formal linguistic analysis on free speech samples from thirty-four schizophrenic patients and eighteen normal controls, matched for age, education and social class. A first 'scan' designated sentences as well-formed or deviant. A second scan identified word-level errors, including neologisms and speech dysfluencies (e.g. pause fillers and false starts). In the third scan grammatical complexity was measured using syntactic tree diagrams that were constructed for each sentence. The fourth scan highlighted grammatical errors. With the aid of a specially developed computer programme, which derived ninety-eight linguistic measures from the data, Morice et al. found that two main types of variable significantly distinguished the schizophrenic and control groups. The first was a set of items relating to reduced speech complexity. The second related to integrity of speech – the schizophrenic patients showed fewer well-formed sentences and more sentences containing both semantic and syntactic errors.

Fraser et al. (1986) repeated essentially the same study on fifty schizophrenic patients and fifty normal controls (and fifty-one manic patients) and again found that the schizophrenic patients had lower scores on the major variables representing complexity of speech, showed fewer well-formed sentences and made more semantic and syntactic errors. Hoffman and Sledge (1988) compared segments of speech from eleven acute admissions with schizophrenia and nine patients with other diagnoses, depression, mania or personality disorder, who were matched for age and education. Unlike the studies of Morice and Ingram (1982) and Fraser et al. (1986), in this study clues to diagnosis were removed from the transcripts and they were analysed under blind conditions. The schizophrenic patients produced nearly three times as many errors as the controls. The major difference was in grammatical errors, and the difference in the rate of semantic errors was slight.

None of these studies examined general intellectual impairment as a possible cause of the differences they found. But this shortcoming pales into insignificance beside another. As Chaika (1990) succinctly put it: 'A major problem in research has been that investigators have not ensured that they were testing only SD [speech disordered] psychotics.' Morice and McNichol (1985) excluded the possibility that the abnormalities were due to drug treatment. Members of Fraser's original group went on to compare speech in acute and chronic patients (King et al., 1990; Thomas et al., 1990), and in patients with positive versus those with negative symptoms (Thomas et al., 1987); and later showed that the same abnormalities were present in patients undergoing their first episode of illness (Thomas et al.,

1996). But these authors almost seem to have gone out of their way to avoid examining the critical question of whether these expressive speech abnormalities were a function of thought disorder.

Chaika (Chaika and Alexander, 1986; see also Chaika, 1990) carried out her own study, comparing the speech of twenty-two thought-disordered patients with twenty-five normal controls. Unfortunately for the present purposes the psychotic sample was not exclusively schizophrenic but included eight patients with mania. Thought disorder was also operationalised somewhat idiosyncratically as presence of one or more of the following: neologising, gibberish, opposite speech, inappropriate rhyming or punning, word salad, inappropriate repetitions/perseverations, faulty cohesion or glossomania. The patients and controls were shown a short video (the 'ice cream story') and immediately afterwards were asked to describe what happened in it. The analysis was largely qualitative, but it found that both the patients and controls produced errors which interrupted the flow of narration. In some cases these took a different form in the two groups. For example, the controls sometimes started a phrase, broke off to insert something, and then resumed, as in:

and then she – her father came home from work, whatever – she asked her father for money.
and a white – it appeared to be white – long-sleeved shirt.

In contrast, when the patients broke off in the middle of a phrase, they never picked it up. These sentences were said as if nothing had been omitted and there was no break in intonation or stress, as in:

what are the and uh there was a scene.
he was blamed for and I didn't think that was fair the way the way they did that either.

Certain types of syntactic error, however, were seen in both groups. For example the normal subjects said:

he charged it *for* her.
it's too close *for* dinnertime.

Whereas the psychotic patients said things like:

two or three minutes *for* get waited on.
there was and when she got home *there was* too near suppertime.
men will try to use you every time for everything *he* wants.

Semantic errors, on the other hand, were found almost exclusively in the psychotic patients. This applied as expected to neologisms, although one control produced a single short stretch of gibberish: 'so therefore she *etuh* she ed she listened'. One patient said 'he twitched through the door', where the intended word was probably switched, as it was a reference to the camera action. Another said 'that's all I can stew' instead of do at the end of a narrative. One manic patient stated that the girl was looking in a trashcan when she was actually looking in a window. Some lexical choices were reminiscent of aphasic phenomena, for example 'The cash register man handled the financial matters' instead of the clerk rang up the sale, and 'he [the father] gets her the coins' instead of he gave her money.

Even this study is not immune to criticism, since, by failing to include a comparison group of non-thought-disordered patients, Chaika and Alexander left open the possibility that some of the errors they found were a feature of schizophrenia in general rather than thought-disordered schizophrenia in particular. Oh *et al.* (2002) closed this final loophole in their study. They collected 200–300 sentences of speech from their six patients with severe thought disorder, the seven without thought disorder and also nine normal individuals who were of a comparable age and estimated IQ distribution to the two patient groups. A number of tasks were used to elicit speech. The first was a ten-minute interview, taken from the 'conversational and expository speech' section of the BDAE. The subjects were then given four pictures and three cartoon stories to describe. They were also asked to tell two fairy stories. The final task was designed to be similar to Chaika's ice cream story: the subjects had to relate what happened in a short computer-animated story about a boy in a toyshop.

Transcripts of the subjects' speech were analysed using Brief Syntactic Analysis (BSA) (Thomas *et al.*, 1996), a simplified form of the linguistic analysis developed by Morice and Ingram (1982). The analysis is performed at the within-sentence analysis, and does not go beyond this to the between-sentence or discourse level. Providing that a sentence is syntactically and semantically well formed, it is not classified as deviant, even if in the context of the discourse it is meaningless. In BSA a sentence is judged syntactically deviant if the rules of syntax are breached, important grammatical structures omitted or if there are structural anomalies. Examples include:

Patient. Then they come in again, and *starts* taking their coats off.
   (*verb disagreement*)
Patient. He goes fishing, and um . . . the ripples by the rock.
   (*missing clause*)

Several types of error can cause a sentence to be rated as semantically deviant in BSA. One type of semantically deviant sentence would be where the meaning was unclear or bizarre because of the way in which particular words were combined within the sentence. For example:

Patient. Seems to be like a white, like a white space deck . . . . . . hand, which is white all over and coloured like a white sort of dome-type hand.
Patient. Is video a wall-pisser?

The second, related type of deviant sentence would be one which contained a word or words that were used in a semantically unacceptable way. For example:

Interviewer. Tell me a bit more about life there.
Patient. Oh, it was superb, you know the trains broke, and the pond fell in the front doorway.

Here, the clause *the pond fell in the front doorway* is semantically deviant because the propositional features of a pond do not allow it to fall in a doorway. If the subject had said the Martian fell in the front doorway this would not have been rated semantically deviant, because, although bizarre, it is conceivable that a Martian could fall in a doorway.

Semantic paraphasias are also rated as semantic errors according to the BSA:

Patient. 'Cause it's [the boat] near the shore and somehow it wouldn't *drown*.

Here, the patient substituted *drown* for *sink* when describing a picture of a seaside scene in which a boat is capsizing.

All sentences identified as deviant were presented to a linguist who was not otherwise involved in the study. They were put in random order with no indication as to whether they came from thought-disordered patients, non-thought-disordered patients or normal controls. The second linguist made a final judgement as to whether the sentence was deviant or not and the form of deviance shown.

The percentage of deviant sentences for each of the patients is shown in Figure 4.2. It can be seen that the thought-disordered patients showed the highest overall proportion of deviant sentences and the control subjects the lowest, with the non-thought-disordered patients being intermediate between the two. Both the thought-disordered and non-thought-disordered patients produced sentences containing syntactic errors in roughly similar proportions (ranges 3.0%–8.3% and 0.5%–7.2% respectively). This rate was generally higher than in the normal controls (range 0.4%–2.7%).

Semantic errors, on the other hand, were greatly over-represented in the thought-disordered group. All of the thought-disordered patients produced some semantically deviant sentences (range 2.5%–7.8%), whereas only three of the non-thought-disordered patients did so, and then only to a lesser degree (range 0%–1.5%). None of the normal controls produced sentences showing this type of deviance.

This study suggests that semantic errors are the characteristic feature of thought disorder, and that syntactic errors are non-specific, a consequence of being schizophrenic rather than showing incoherent speech. The measures of dysfluency and sentence complexity in BSA were also found to be non-specific, being approximately equally distributed between the thought-disordered and the non-thought-disordered patients. There was also little to suggest that the tendency to make semantic and syntactic errors in schizophrenia was a function of general

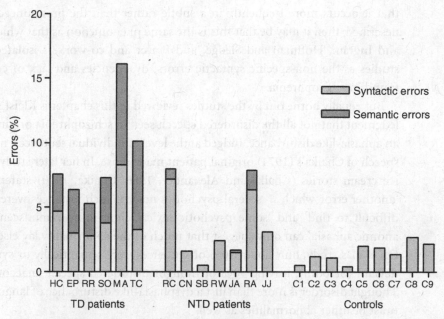

Figure 4.2   Errors in expressed speech in thought-disordered and non-thought-disordered schizophrenic patients and normal controls (from Oh *et al.*, 2002)

intellectual impairment. Thus, in Figure 4.2, the patients' scores are ordered from left to right in the same increasing order of overall intellectual impairment as in the earlier part of the study; there is no evidence that either form of error increases as intellectual function becomes more impaired.

Conclusion

It appears that the heretical and deviationist Kleist was right all along: language abnormality does make a contribution to the phenomenon of thought disorder in schizophrenia. If one wished to construe this language disturbance as a form of dysphasia, then it would be one which was characterised chiefly by semantic errors in expressed speech. if, on the other hand, one wanted to distance oneself from this view, one could point to the lack of an obvious comprehension deficit and the preserved naming, both of which mark 'schizophasia' out as different from most if not all known forms of fluent dysphasia.

Kleist also described an additional form of dysphasia-like disturbance in schizophrenia. This was agrammatism, a simplification and coarsening of sentence structure, essentially similar to Broca's aphasia, which occurred particularly in catatonic patients and was associated with lack of spontaneity. If, as Kleist implied, this form of language disturbance is unrelated to thought disorder, and assuming that it occurs more frequently in a subtle rather than the pronounced form he described, then it may be that this is the same phenomenon as that which Morice and Ingram, Hoffman and Sledge, and Fraser and co-workers isolated in their studies as the non-specific syntactic errors, dysfluencies and lack of complexity found in schizophrenia.

But equally borne out by the studies reviewed in this chapter is Kleist's acknowledgment that not all the disordered speech seen in schizophrenia originates from an aphasia-like disturbance. Judged at the level of individual sentences, most of the speech of Chaika's (1974) original patient made sense. In her later study using the ice cream stories (Chaika and Alexander, 1986; Chaika, 1990) statements like 'another error which . . . several psychotics made', 'such instances were not at all difficult to find' and 'some psychotic lexical choices are reminiscent of mild anomic aphasia' can only suggest that much of the abnormality lay elsewhere. In Oh *et al.*'s study, only about 10% of sentences were semantically or syntactically deviant (or both), leaving 90% of thought-disordered speech unaccounted for. Thought disorder is more than just a dysphasia-like disturbance of language; there must be other abnormalities as well.

5

Thought disorder and communicative competence

There is more to making one's self understood than knowing the meaning of words and the rules that govern how words (and the sounds that make them up) are put together. What is also required is the ability to use language effectively for the purposes of communication, a skill broadly referred to as 'communicative competence'. Three forms of knowledge are relevant to this. The first includes the range of devices which enable speakers to communicate stretches of speech longer than a single sentence; this is referred to as discourse knowledge. The second is the shared knowledge that speakers and listeners have, which allows them to interpret aspects of meaning over and above the literal meaning of the words themselves; this is part of the area of linguistics known as pragmatics. The third subdivision of communicative competence forms the subject matter of another area of linguistics, that of sociolinguistics. Sociolinguistic knowledge covers the social conventions associated with the language one speaks, including knowing how to use language in different social situations, and how to adjust one's register depending on who one is communicating with.

Communicative competence develops gradually in children, and a rough idea of the importance of discourse and pragmatic knowledge in conversation can be gained from samples of speech from very young children. Hoff (2001) provided this example of a three-year-old who was asked to make up a story, and replied 'A little duck went swimming. Then a crab came. A lobster came. And a popsicle was playing by itself.' The individual sentences are correctly formed, and by and large the ideas expressed are understandable. But taken as a whole, the story fails to make sense. Young children also fail to abide by sociolinguistic conventions, such as politeness, but this does not compromise the intelligibility of speech in the same way, although it may cause embarrassment.

The possibility of understanding thought disorder in this way was not lost on some early authors. These included no less a figure than Piaget, who suggested that the child's thinking lay midway between the autistic thinking of the schizophrenic patient and the logical thought of the adult; and Vygotsky, who suggested that thinking in schizophrenia reversed the normal ontological development of thinking. However, it was another author who spelled out the potential similarities most clearly:

The young child, Piaget finds, takes it for granted that he will be understood and is astonished when, after giving a hopelessly inadequate rendition of a story for example, he discovers that his hearer has not grasped the relationships that he himself certainly felt were implied. Moreover there is a curious lack in the children's talk of that order and sequence one is accustomed to find in adult narrative or exposition; and there is an outstanding absence of causal links. In the explanation he gives, the child evidently 'feels' that certain things belong together; but he does not make this connection in any way explicit. He simply juxtaposes related material in whatever order it happens to occur, instead of arranging it in a natural or logical order and connecting it by explicit causal links. He is apparently unable to place himself in the position of others, to imagine their points of view and so to realize their needs and his own gaps. The end result is that in place of well-integrated concepts that can be expressed in a conventional form and thus used as a common currency for communication between individuals, there is a loose conglomerate personally quite satisfying to the as-yet asocial child, but failing in what should be its essential characteristic – communicability.

This author was Cameron (1938) describing the background to the study presented in Chapter 1, in which he originally set out to test the hypothesis that thought disorder represented a regression to childish modes of reasoning. However, when he gave his thought-disordered patients simple causal sentences to complete (a technique he borrowed from a study by Piaget), he found that the kind of reasoning they showed was typical of adults, and there was no evidence of an excess of the types of responses typically used by young children.[1]

At the time Cameron rejected the view that schizophrenic speech represented a regression to a more primitive pattern seen in young children. Fifty years on, the idea that thought disorder could represent a breakdown in communicative competence is a thriving area of research. Three areas in particular have received attention, two of which are considered aspects of pragmatics – failure to make use of context and failure to take account of the needs of the listener. The third concerns the possibility that patients with thought disorder show a failure at the level of discourse, specifically a lack of cohesion in connected speech.

Thought disorder as failure to make use of context

By common agreement, pragmatics covers the broad range of topics listed in Box 5.1. While it is difficult to imagine how many of these, such as speech acts, deixis, presuppositions and entailments could be relevant to thought disorder, it is quite possible to entertain the notion that incoherent schizophrenic speech is incoherent

---

[1] Nearly 70% of the responses fell into the two adult categories of cause and effect and logical justification, and there was nothing like the over 80% preponderance of responses invoking psychological motivation typically seen in six-year-old children.

because of a failure to take context into account. In linguistics, 'context' refers to the actual linguistic material (also known as co-text) or to the physical surroundings in which the utterance is made (usually referred to as just context). Yule (1996) illustrates with this example:

(a) The cheese sandwich is made with white bread.
(b) The cheese sandwich just left without paying.

In both these utterances, the meaning of 'the cheese sandwich' is identifiable through the linguistic material that follows. In (a) the co-text tells us that an edible substance is being spoken of, whereas in (b) a person (or at least something that is animate and not made of bread) is being referred to. However, we depend also on physical context – the physical surroundings of the speaker and listener when the utterance is made – to confirm our interpretation of these and other utterances. In both cases, especially in (b) where figurative language is being used, failure to provide such contextual material could make it difficult to follow what the speaker was saying.

Box 5.1 Pragmatics

(From Yule, 1996; Thomas, 1995; Levinson, 1983)

Pragmatics is a slippery term to define, and indeed its precise definition and the areas it does or does not cover are matters still discussed by linguists. Various definitions exist, but there are at least four (closely related) aspects of language that have come to be generally accepted as falling under its heading. These are:

- The study of speaker meaning – that is, what the speaker intends to say or mean by his utterance, over and above what the words within that utterance might mean by themselves. For example, the utterance 'I am cold' – taken literally – is a declarative statement about one's temperature. However, it could also be a request for the window to be shut, depending on the speaker's intention. How the speaker's intention is recognised depends on many factors, including knowledge of the cooperative principle and implicature ('additional conveyed meaning', related closely to communicating more than is being said below, see also Grice's maxims in main text). The speaker's communicative intention will also determine the kind of speech act – actions performed by utterances, such as apologies, compliments or threats – used.
- The study of contextual meaning – that is, how context (linguistic and physical) influences meaning and what is said. For example, a statement overheard at a party 'The Pearsons are on coke', could mean one of three things: that they are drinking Coca-Cola, that they use cocaine or that they have solid fuel heating.

Box 5.1 (cont.)

What the words actually meant on that occasion (and the speaker's intention) can only be determined by the context.

- The study of how more gets communicated than is said – we have already seen how an utterance has 'unsaid' parts to it. Included in these unsaid aspects are presuppositions and entailments: two aspects of information that are treated as known, and therefore not generally stated. In addition, extra-linguistic information about the speaker can sometimes be communicated. Yule uses the example of answering to the question 'How are you?' when among different linguistic communities. In an English-speaking community, a simple 'Fine' or 'Well' would be the norm but answering that way in an Arabic-speaking community would tell the listener that you were an outsider (a more conventional answer would be a phrase that meant 'Allah be praised'). Inference is an important process that listeners use to help them interpret these unsaid aspects of information.

- The study of the expression of relative distance (deixis) – that is, the speaker's decision on how close (physically, socially or conceptually) to the listener they are, which will determine how much to say and to leave out. Saying 'Each person has to clean up after him or herself' as opposed to 'Somebody didn't clean up after himself' creates a distance between the speaker and listener, where a potentially personal statement becomes an impersonal one. Similarly, saying 'We clean up after ourselves around here' implies that this rule applies to the speaker as well. Deictic expressions can be personal ('you', 'me'), temporal ('now') or spatial ('here').

Something very close to a failure to make use of linguistic context (i.e. co-text) was the centrepiece of a theory of thought disorder suggested by Chapman and co-workers (Chapman *et al.*, 1964; Chapman and Chapman, 1973). Their proposal was that schizophrenic patients showed a bias towards the strong or preferred meaning of a word even when the context dictated otherwise. One consequence of such a bias would be that the speaker would find it more difficult than normal speakers to prevent the strong meaning of a word from intruding into speech, no matter what the context. They cited one of Bleuler's (1911) patients who enumerated the members of her family as 'father, son,' and then added 'and the Holy Ghost'. The same difficulty could also cause them to misinterpret words in conversation. Thus, another of Bleuler's patients replied to the question 'Is something weighing heavily on your mind?' with 'Yes, iron is heavy.' – he chose the literal meaning 'weigh' despite a context which indicated that a figurative meaning was intended.

Chapman *et al.* (1964) tested their hypothesis by requiring schizophrenic patients to interpret words in context. They prepared two sets of nineteen sentences containing words whose context pointed either to its strong meaning or to a non-preferred weaker meaning, followed by multiple choice alternatives, for example:

Robert said he likes rare meat.
This means:

A. He likes the kind of meat that is exceedingly uncommon.
B. He likes a meat with bones in it.
C. He likes partially cooked meat.

He couldn't find bear meat because it was rare.
This means:

A. It was meat with bones in it.
B. It was an exceedingly uncommon meat.
C. It was partially cooked meat.

The test was administered to a group of chronic schizophrenic patients and normal controls matched for age, education and verbal IQ. The prediction was that the schizophrenic patients would make more errors than controls when the weaker meaning was required. This was supported: the patients made significantly more errors than the controls, choosing the strong meaning of the word when the context suggested the weaker one. However, they also made significantly more errors than the controls when the correct choice was the stronger meaning of the word, but here Chapman *et al.* were able to demonstrate that these errors were mainly on words where there was some uncertainty as to which was the weaker or stronger meaning.

Chapman and Chapman (1973) were among the earliest advocates of the need to control for the tendency to general poor performance found in schizophrenia, but the evidence they provided that their finding did not reflect this was distinctly limited. Also, although Chapman and Chapman were specifically interested in abnormal response bias as a possible explanation of thought disorder, they did not examine groups of patients with and without the symptom. Some subsequent studies replicated Chapman *et al.*'s (1964) original finding that schizophrenic patients are biased toward the strongest meaning, no matter what the context (Benjamin and Watt, 1969; Mourer, 1971; Roberts and Schuham, 1974), but others failed to do so (Blaney, 1974; Neuringer *et al.*, 1969; Miller, 1974). None of these studies were a methodological advance on Chapman *et al.*'s original study in either of these respects.

A lengthy hiatus then followed, during which schizophrenia research occupied itself solely with context in its general sense, rather than in the more restricted sense of surrounding linguistic material. This took the form of an exploration of context effects using the Continuous Performance Test. This is a vigilance test in which subjects see a long series of letters on a screen and have to respond each time a certain one appears. In a variant of the task, the subjects have to respond only when the target letter follows another one, which provides the 'context'. These studies may or may not have provided evidence for 'a degradation in the internal representation of context' in schizophrenia (see Cohen and Servan-Schreiber, 1992), but they have never attempted to relate this to thought disorder or any other symptom.

A return to linguistic context – and its relationship to thought disorder – has recently been marked by a study by Kuperberg *et al.* (1998). They examined the effects of context in a word monitoring task developed by Tyler (1992), in which normal individuals show a progressive increase in reaction time to recognise target words presented in sentences that violate the normal rules of pragmatics, semantics and syntax. Their subjects were twenty-seven patients selected on the basis of an initial screening interview as showing either marked thought disorder ($N = 17$) or no evidence of this ($N = 10$). This was determined using the Thought, Language and Communication Index (Liddle, 1995), a scale similar to Andreasen's TLC scale, in which a series of pictures is used to elicit disordered speech. There were also ten normal controls matched for age, education and estimated premorbid IQ.

The subjects were given one of a series of target nouns, such as *guitar*, and then listened to pairs of pre-recorded sentences through headphones. The first sentence provided a minimal and not highly constraining context for the second sentence. The target word was in the second sentence and this was either linguistically acceptable, or violated pragmatic, semantic or syntactic rules. Some examples of the violations are shown in Table 5.1. The subjects were instructed to press a key as soon as they heard the target word. The onset of each target word triggered a timing device that measured the delay in responding.

Kuperberg *et al.*'s findings are shown in Figure 5.1. The normal subjects' reaction time to identify the target words showed a progressive increase as the violation moved from pragmatic, to semantic, to syntactically anomalous sentences. In other words as the linguistic violation became more marked, they were increasingly unable to make use of the advantage afforded by the context of the preceding word to anticipate the target word and respond quickly. Thus reaction time was slowed slightly when the violation was pragmatic, i.e. when the sentence still made some sense; was greater for semantic violations, i.e. when the sentence no longer made literal sense; and was greater still when the sentence violated syntactic rules and the expectation that the target word would follow was least. The non-thought-disordered patients were generally slower than the normal controls, but showed a similar progressive increase in reaction time across the conditions. However, the thought-disordered patients showed a flatter pattern – despite having generally longer

Table 5.1 Types of linguistic violations in Kuperberg *et al.*'s study

(From Kuperberg *et al.*, 1998)

Linguistic violation	Explanation	Example
None	Baseline condition against which the other conditions are evaluated.	'The crowd was waiting eagerly; the young man grabbed the guitar...'
Pragmatic	The verb preceding the target is replaced by another verb of the same frequency. This makes the sentence pragmatically implausible with respect to our knowledge of real world events.	'The crowd was waiting eagerly; the young man buried the guitar...'
Semantic	Verbs are selected so that their semantic properties are incompatible with the semantic properties of the noun.	'The crowd was waiting eagerly; the young man drank the guitar...'
Syntactic*	Intransitive verbs are chosen that cannot be followed by a noun in direct object position.	'The crowd was waiting eagerly; the young man slept the guitar...'

Note: * In this condition, the violation was referred to as syntactic. However, it should be noted that it was also a semantic and/or pragmatic violation. Indeed, all the stimuli were hierarchically organised; that is, the semantic anomaly was also a pragmatic anomaly, and the syntactic anomaly was also a semantic anomaly.

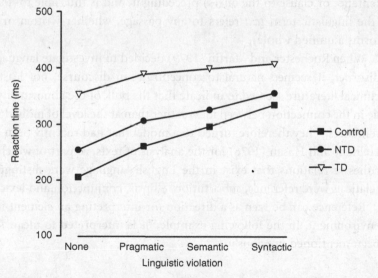

Figure 5.1   Effects of different types of linguistic violation on reaction time to target words in thought-disordered and non-thought-disordered schizophrenic patients and normal subjects (from Kuperberg *et al.*, 1998, American Psychological Association. Reprinted with permission)

reaction times than the non-thought-disordered patients the different linguistic violations appeared to have little effect.

Kuperberg *et al.* concluded that patients with thought disorder fail to use linguistic context to process speech on-line, that is while they are comprehending it. They went on to argue that the ability to use linguistic context on-line is also necessary for speech production, where it guides the retrieval of appropriate words for subsequent parts of an utterance or series of utterances. A failure here could lead to the intrusion of inappropriate words into the flow of speech. Whether or not this argument is accepted, Kuperberg *et al.*'s study takes Chapman and Chapman's context theory of thought disorder a step forward and so advances the general cause for the involvement of a disturbance of communicability.

Thought disorder as lack of cohesion in discourse

When a person is presented with a piece of speech spanning more than one sentence, he or she can usually tell whether those sentences are related to one another or are just a random collection of sentences. This is because of the cohesive devices that the sentences contain. Such cohesive devices are evident in the first sentence of this very paragraph. By using the word *those* in 'he or she can usually tell whether those sentences are related to one another . . . ' it has been indicated to the reader that the sentences being written about are the ones in the 'piece of speech' referred to in the preceding clause. In this way, the reader is able to link a sentence or clause to the one(s) preceding it, and is thus able to 'follow' the text (the linguistic term *text* refers to any passage, whether written or spoken, that forms a unified whole).

When Rochester and Martin (1979) decided to investigate language in thought disorder, it seemed natural to concentrate on discourse, not least because the clinical literature seemed to indicate that the bulk of the abnormality appeared to lie in the connection between ideas rather than at the level of individual words and sentences. They therefore turned to a model that had recently been developed by Halliday and Hasan (1976) for the analysis of texts, as part of which five types of cohesive relations that exist in the English language were distinguished. These relations were reference, substitution, ellipsis, conjunction and lexical cohesion.[2]

Reference can be seen as a direction for interpreting an element in terms of its environment. In the following example, *he* is interpreted to mean *John*, who has been mentioned previously.

---

[2] Halliday and and Hasan (1976) were careful to emphasise that this classification of cohesive relations should not be seen as a rigid division into 'watertight compartments', and acknowledged that there are instances of cohesion that lie on the borderline between two types.

John was my best friend at school. *He* taught me how to climb trees.

In English, personals (*he*, *she*, *they*, etc.), demonstratives (*this*, *that*, etc.) and comparatives (*smaller than*, *equal to*, *same*, etc.) make up reference items.

Substitution can be thought of as the replacement of one item by another, as in:

I like your dress. Is it a new *one*?

Here, *one* is a substitute for *dress*. Only the items *one(s)*, *same*, *do*, *so*, and *not* can occur as substitutes.

Put simply, ellipsis can be defined as substitution by zero. It occurs when something that is structurally necessary is left unsaid, for example:

Do you have a light? Yes, I have.

Utterances that did not make use of ellipsis and substitution would appear stilted and unusually formal, or else signal to the listener that there was some significance in repeating what could have been left out.

The fourth type of cohesive relation is conjunction. There are four types of conjunctive relations, each expressing a different relationship: additive, adversative, causal and temporal. An example of each is shown below.

She worked all day, almost without stopping.

(a) *And* in all this time, no one offered her a drink. (additive)
(b) *Yet* she was not aware of being tired. (adversative)
(c) *So* by the time she finished, she was tired. (causal)
(d) *Then*, when it got dark, she stopped. (temporal)

Lexical cohesion is the cohesive effect achieved by the selection of vocabulary. This can be achieved in two ways, reiteration and collocation. Reiteration is a form of lexical cohesion which involves (at one end of the scale) the repetition of a lexical item, the use of a general word to refer back to a lexical item (at the other end of the scale), and, in between, the use of a synonym, near-synonym or superordinate. This is illustrated below in an example from Halliday and Hasan (1976):

I turned to the ascent of the peak.

(a) The *ascent* was perfectly easy. (same word)
(b) The *climb* was perfectly easy. (synonym)
(c) The *task* was perfectly easy. (superordinate)
(d) The *thing* was perfectly easy. (general word)

Cohesion can also be achieved through collocation, or the association of pairs of words that regularly co-occur. The cohesive effect of such pairs is achieved more by their tendency to share the same lexical environment, i.e. to occur in collocation with each other. This category includes pairs of opposites, such as complement-aries (*boy – girl, stand up – sit down*), antonyms (*love – hate, wet – dry*) and converses (*order – obey*). It would also include pairs of words drawn from the same ordered series (*Tuesday – Thursday*), or unordered lexical sets (*road – rail, red – green*). These pairs often stand in some recognisable lexicosemantic relation with each other. However, there is also the possibility of cohesion between any pair of lexical items that are some way associated with each other in the language, but whose meaning relation is not easy to classify in systematic semantic terms (e.g. *laugh – joke, blade – sharp*). In general, any two lexical items tending to appear in similar contexts (having the same collocation patterns) will generate a cohesive force if they occur in adjacent sentences. Cohesion achieved through this sort of lexical relationship is not limited to pairs of words; it is possible also for long cohesive chains to occur (*poetry . . . literature . . . reader . . . writer . . . style*).

Rochester and Martin (1979) selected groups of ten patients with thought disorder and ten without from a larger sample of 40 acute admissions meeting an early set of diagnostic criteria for schizophrenia (the New Haven Schizophrenia Index). Presence or absence of thought disorder was decided on the basis of videotaped interviews, which were assessed by two psychiatrists who were not otherwise involved in the study. The two groups were both relatively young, averagely educated, acutely ill patients and they did not differ significantly in age, years of education and IQ. A group of ten normal controls was also recruited; these subjects were on average older and better educated, and they also had a higher IQ.

Speech was obtained in three settings: an unstructured interview lasting about half an hour; a brief narrative, which the subjects had to retell after it was read to them; and a task requiring them to describe cartoon pictures. Rochester and Martin (1979) then applied the analysis of cohesion to transcripts of the speech. For this, they selected two sections of about fifteen independent clauses each from the interviews, plus the full text of the narratives (the speech from the cartoon description task was not included in this part of the study). This amounted to approximately 300 clauses per group. Each clause contained on average 2.6 cohesive links to other clauses, giving an overall database of 3,100 observations in all three groups together. Each cohesive tie was indicated in the transcripts while listening to the recordings, and the category it fell into was noted. In order to check reliability, a second assessor carried out the same exercise on three subjects in each group. The reliability ranged from 95–100% in the interviews and 87–100% for the narratives. There was almost complete agreement on the type of cohesive tie.

The findings for the overall number of ties used by the three groups are shown in Table 5.2a. The normal speakers used significantly more cohesive ties than both groups of schizophrenic speakers. In narratives the rate was almost double; in interviews the difference was less marked. However, there were no significant differences between the thought-disordered and non-thought-disordered patients. The findings were similar when ties/clause was used as a measure, which corrected for minor differences in the overall numbers of clauses the three groups produced in some of the conditions.

As can be seen in Table 5.2b, there were also no great differences in the proportion of four different ties used by the three groups (substitution accounted for less than 1% of the ties and so was not examined). The only significant effect concerned lexical cohesion, where the thought-disordered patients were in fact found to use more ties of this type than the non-thought-disordered patients, although neither group differed significantly from the controls.

Table 5.2 Amount of cohesion in schizophrenic patients with and without thought disorder and normal subjects

(From Rochester and Martin, 1979, reproduced with permission)

(a) Overall cohesion

	Ties per clause	
	Narrative*	Interview
TD patients	2.61	2.04
NTD patients	2.95	1.97
Normal subjects	3.86	2.27

Note: * One-way ANOVA $F_{(2,27)} = 7.2$, $P < 0.005$; TD, NTD < Normal.

(b) Percentage of ties per category

	Reference	Conjunction	Lexical cohesion	Ellipsis
Narrative				
TD patients	52.0	21.7	24.9	0.7
NTD patients	49.9	24.1	22.8	3.2
Normal subjects	46.5	21.1	30.3	2.0
Interview				
TD	28.6	20.2	45.8*	4.0
NTD	33.8	25.9	31.3	8.1
Normal	29.9	28.1	36.0	5.8

Note: * One-way ANOVA $F_{(2,27)} = 3.83$, $P < 0.05$; NTD < TD, but neither significantly different from normal subjects.

Thus far, Rochester and Martin's results pointed to a reduction in the use of cohesive ties in schizophrenia, but they had found nothing relating specifically to thought disorder. However, they then went on to investigate not just the number of ties, but the way in which schizophrenic patients used them. In order to do this they selected one particular class of cohesive tie, reference – where a personal pronoun (he, she, they, etc.), a demonstrative (this, that, etc.) or a comparative (smaller than, equal to, etc.) is used to replace a noun or a proper noun. The reference system allows speakers to mark out directions for listeners, enabling them to identify participants referred to in the discourse. In normal discourse, speakers constantly remind their listeners about the shared knowledge between them at the same time as they are introducing new information. For example, once a participant has been introduced in a text, the speaker subsequently uses reference to remind the listener of this knowledge by use of a definite article or pronoun. If, however, an individual incorrectly reminds the listener, indicating that a referent has already been given when in fact it has not, the listener might well find the speaker difficult to follow.

Rochester and Martin illustrated this with the following example of a thought-disordered patient relating the Donkey and the Salt story:[3]

(1) A donkey was carrying salt/ (2) and *he* went through a river/ (3) and he decided to go for a swim/ (4) and his salt started dissolving off of him into the water/ (5) and it did/ (6) it left him hanging there/ (7) so he crawled out on the other side and became a mastodon/ (8) *it* gets unfrozen/ (9) it's up in the Arctic right now/ (10) it's a block of ice/ (11) and a block of ice gets planted in/ (12) it's forced into a square right? (13) ever studied that sort of a formation, block of ice in the ground?/ (14) well, it fights the perma frost/ (15) it pushes it away/ (16) and lets things go up around *it*/ (17) you can see they're like, *they're* almost like a pattern with a flower/ (18) *they* start from the middle/ (19) and it's like a submerged ice cube/(20) that got frozen into the soil afterwards / . . . .

Although in (2) the patient initially correctly reminded the listener that, by using 'he', he was referring to the donkey, in (17) and (18) there were no obvious candidate referents for 'they're' and 'they'. There were also a number of other instances where what was being referred to was not readily accessible, for example 'it' in (8) and (16).

Rochester and Martin carried out an analysis of reference on all of the three types of speech they collected (unstructured interview, retelling a story, describing cartoons). This analysis was not easy for anyone other than a linguist to

---

[3] A donkey, loaded with salt had to wade a stream. He fell down and for a few minutes lay comfortably in the cool water. When he got up, he felt relieved of a great part of his burden, because the salt had dissolved in the water. The donkey took note of this advantage and applied it the following day when, this time loaded with sponges, he again went through the same stream. This time he fell purposely, but was grossly deceived. The sponges soaked up the water and were considerably heavier than before. The burden was so great that he fell and could not go on (or drowned in some versions).

understand, and was also highly complicated in its own right. The main finding was that the thought-disordered subjects showed more instances of unclear reference compared with both the non-thought-disordered patients and the normal controls. However, whether there were statistically significant differences between the two patient groups is virtually impossible to reconstruct from the data they presented.

Rochester and Martin's general finding that schizophrenic speakers use fewer cohesive ties than normal speakers was not replicated in at least two further studies. Using interviews to elicit speech, Harvey (1983) found no overall decrease in the number of cohesive ties used by schizophrenic speakers. Chaika and Lambe (1989) also failed to find differences in the overall number of cohesive ties between thought-disordered schizophrenic patients and normal controls in a narrative task (the ice cream stories described in Chapter 4).

In contrast, these studies were consistent in finding evidence for unclear reference in patients with thought disorder. In his study, Harvey (1983) reported that his thought-disordered patients used 'significantly fewer implicit references and significantly more unclear, ambiguous and generic references than did NTD patients'. Harvey's thought-disordered group consisted of ten schizophrenic and ten manic patients, but no significant difference was found between the two in terms of reference performance. Chaika and Lambe (1989) noted that five of the twenty-two patients in their study, all of whom were thought-disordered (but eight of whom had a diagnosis of mania rather than schizophrenia), showed inappropriate reference, for example saying 'she' without an antecedent and with no reference to characters in the story. This was not seen at all in the controls.

Using their own communication disturbances index which rates speech for reference failures (as well as ambiguous word meaning and structural unclarities), Docherty and her colleagues (Docherty et al., 1996; Docherty and Gottesman, 2000) have also consistently found reference abnormalities in the speech of schizophrenic patients. This group of studies, however, was concerned with a different set of questions, and so the presence of thought disorder was not always specified. Nevertheless, in those studies where thought disorder was rated (Docherty et al., 1988; Docherty and Gordinier, 1999; Docherty et al., 2003), it was found to be significantly correlated with the presence of referential disturbances.[4]

Oh et al. (unpublished data from their 2002 study) also investigated cohesive ties in their study, described in the last chapter, of six schizophrenic patients with thought disorder and seven without the symptom. As in the within-sentence analysis, nine normal control subjects were included. The use of the single-case study

---

[4] In Docherty et al.'s (2003) paper, the components of 'referential disturbance' that were found to be significantly correlated with thought disorder were confused references and ambiguous word meaning, but not the other types of referential disturbance (vague references, missing information references, wrong word references).

approach allowed the authors to analyse a larger corpus of speech than the average of thirty to forty clauses per subject in Rochester and Martin's (1979) study. One hundred sentences from each subject were scanned for the five categories of cohesion. Each instance of cohesion, that is, the occurrence of a pair of cohesively related items, was called a tie. As it seemed likely that the number of cohesive devices used by the schizophrenic patients might be less interesting than the way in which they were used, errors or non-conventional use of cohesive devices were also identified. This applied to all classes of tie, not just reference, and was determined on the basis of a clear breach of linguistic rules. The criteria for scoring an error are shown in Table 5.3. In rare cases where there was some ambiguity about whether an error should be scored or not it was counted as normal.

The schizophrenic patients collectively produced fewer cohesive ties than the controls (mean 133.9 ($SD = 26.18$) vs. 161.0 ($SD = 32.34$) ties/subject). This difference was not significant, although it should be remembered that the number of subjects in each group was small. There was also no significant difference between the thought-disordered and non-thought-disordered patients in the average number of cohesive ties (126.2 ($SD = 10.21$) vs. 140.6 ($SD = 15.55$) ties/subject). The thought-disordered and non-thought-disordered schizophrenic patients did not differ in the number of ties used in any category. A significant difference, however, was found between the schizophrenic patients as a group and the healthy controls, the patients using fewer reference and conjunction ties.

In contrast to the findings for numbers of ties, the schizophrenic patients as a group made significantly more errors than the normal speakers (total 99 vs. 4, respectively). As shown in Table 5.4, the errors were strikingly over-represented in the thought-disordered patients. It is also evident that the differences were almost wholly restricted to two categories, reference and lexical cohesion.[5]

This last finding has an intriguing postscript. According to Halliday and Hasan (1976) the five cohesive devices can be categorised as semantic or structural. For example, reference is a semantic relation and it is an indication that meaning can be retrieved from elsewhere in the text, though not necessarily in the form of the actual word or words required. The four types of conjunctive relations (see above) also each express a different semantic relationship between the sentences linked. Lexical cohesive items create links between sentences through the lexico-semantic relationship that exists between and among words. In contrast, substitution and ellipsis both denote a relation between structural items. Their function is to cohere

---

[5] Ragin and Oltmanns (1986) compared lexical cohesion during and after psychotic episodes in speech obtained from schizophrenic, manic and schizoaffective patients with FTD. They also found an association between thought disorder and lexical cohesion: elevated or excessive lexical cohesion was present when schizophrenic patients were thought disordered, but decreased after the psychotic phase.

Table 5.3 Criteria for rating ties as erroneous in Oh *et al.*'s (2002) study

Cohesive tie	Criterion for error	Example
Reference	If referent was ambiguous, not in text, or wrong pronoun (e.g. wrong gender, singular instead of plural) was used.	But uh ... my father was not a machine, my father wasn't a machine | but ... he got <u>him</u> from a ... a little baby inside a capsule
Substitution and ellipsis	If word or phrase structure that substitution or elliptical devices replaced could not be explicitly identified (one of the conditions of subsitution and ellipsis).	
Conjunction	If semantic relation that conjunctive device is signifying is obviously wrong e.g. 'and' used instead of 'but'.	It's a picture of a circus ring. | <u>But</u> the ring master is in it.
Lexical cohesion	An error was recorded if the second word of the pair occurring in the adjacent sentence did not contribute to the cohesiveness, or appeared in a sentence that did not follow from the previous one.	When people who come in here shouldn't try to get out, we ought to be locked up, and put into ... a pair of hand*cuffs*! Where do you get your <u>cuff</u> links from?

Note: \| = sentence boundary.

one piece of text to another using the actual words and/or structures present in the text. Even at the between-sentence level, this study suggests that it is semantic abnormality which defines the expressive speech of schizophrenic patients.

Taking into account the listener's needs: Grice's Maxims and Theory of Mind

It was Grice who first developed a theory of how conversation works, particularly why it is that we are able to converse effectively, even though much of what we mean is not expressed directly by our actual words. He drew a distinction between

Table 5.4 Number of errors (per hundred sentences) for each of the cohesion categories in thought-disordered and non-thought-disordered patients

(From Oh *et al.*, 2002)

Cohesive category	TD patients						NTD patients						
	HC	EP	RR	SO	MA	TC	RC	CN	SB	RW	JA	RA	JJ
Reference	2	9	12	13	7	8	–	–	1	–	2	1	1
Substitution	–	–	–	–	–	–	–	–	–	–	–	–	–
Ellipsis	1	–	–	–	–	1	–	–	–	–	–	–	–
Conjunction	–	–	–	–	–	–	–	–	–	–	–	–	–
Lexical cohesion	2	–	12	10	14	3	–	–	–	–	–	–	–

what is actually said and what is, in his term, implicated. This distinction is illustrated in the following example taken from Malmkjaer (1991):

A and B are talking about a mutual friend C, who is now working in a bank. A asks B how C is getting on in his job, and B replies, 'Oh quite well I think; he likes his colleagues, and he hasn't been to prison yet.'

What is implicated (and unsaid) here depends on many facts about A, B and C, and their life histories. Part of the reason conversation participants are able to cope with implicatures in speech (although they are left unsaid) is because these participants are adhering to a principle of cooperativeness. According to Grice, being cooperative involves adhering to the following four maxims (Grice, 1957, 1975):[6]

(a) Quantity (contribution should be as informative as is necessary for a successful exchange, and not overly informative)
(b) Quality (speaker's contributions ought to be true)
(c) Relevance (contributions should be relevant to the purpose of the exchange)
(d) Manner (contribution should be perspicuous – it should be orderly, brief, avoiding obscurity and ambiguity).

The mutual adherence by participants to Gricean Maxims (the cooperative principle) means that when a listener is confronted by a sentence that does not make literal sense, he knows that something meaningful must have been intended. He then tries to recover the non-literal meaning from context, shared knowledge and so on. In other words, by combining the literal meaning of an utterance, the analysis of its context and the assumption of the co-operative nature of conversation, the listener is able to work out what is really being said.

---

[6] Clark and Haviland (1977) have added the maxim of Antecedence, which dictates 'that speakers must construct utterances so that listeners only have one direct antecedent for any given piece of information'.

Grice's maxims did not only explain how listeners derive meaning from what is unsaid, they were also an acknowledgment of the listener's needs in conversation, and it was not long before they were applied to thought disorder. Initially, Buckingham (1982) proposed that patients with the symptom might be flouting Gricean maxims – which Grice himself recognised that normal individuals also do – but doing it to such an extent that the listener got lost. According to Grice, normal individuals regularly flout maxims, but they do so in such a way that their listeners can normally make 'bridges' or 'links' and thereby draw the intended inference. For example, people flout the maxim of quality (not saying what one believes to be untrue or lacks evidence) when being ironic, sarcastic, or exaggerating. Providing a prospective department chairman with uncalled for detail about how good a staff member's teaching was, thus violating the maxim of quantity (i.e. be only as informative as the current purposes require), could allow the chairman to draw the inference that the person concerned did not publish very much. Similarly, ambiguity and obscurity may be introduced into a conversation (thus violating the maxim of manner) for dramatic effect or to alert the listener to potentially important information. It could be that schizophrenic patients took this flouting to the extreme, leaving the listener too many bridges to span, though not deliberately. Or, as Buckingham put it, 'the patients fail to take the view of the listener into account, but the failure does not appear to be purposeful'.

The baton then passed to Frith (1992), whose first step was to flesh out the argument. He took as his starting point a study by Cohen (Cohen and Camhi, 1967; Cohen, 1978) in which both schizophrenic and non-schizophrenic subjects took the role of either speaker or listener. The speaker had to describe a coloured disc in such a way that the listener could pick it out from a number of other slightly different coloured ones. When the schizophrenic patients took the role of the listener they had no difficulty in using the information they received to select the correct disc. However, they performed significantly more poorly in the role of speaker.[7] This apparent problem with using language for the purpose of communication led to a discussion of Gricean maxims, pragmatics and the requirement for successful communication 'to take account of the knowledge, beliefs, and intentions of the person to whom we are speaking'. After bringing in Rochester and Martin's (1979) arguments about the need for adequate referents and cohesive ties in discourse, Frith finally arrived at the following position:

My conclusion is that some schizophrenic 'thought disorder' reflects a disorder of communication, caused in part by a failure of the patient to take account of the listener's knowledge in

---

[7] Children aged four and five are also not very successful in similar sorts of task; when asked to describe one item in an array of objects so that a visually separated listener with the same array could identify the item referred to, they provided clues like 'Daddy's shirt', which were not helpful to the listener (Glucksberg et al., 1975).

formulating their speech. This theory explains the asymmetry observed by Cohen, that schizophrenics could understand normals, but normals could not understand schizophrenics. The normal speaker takes account of the listener's lack of knowledge, and thus the schizophrenic listener can understand. The schizophrenic speaker does *not* take account of the listener's lack of knowledge, and thus the listener has difficulty in understanding.

By this point Frith's argument had moved beyond Gricean maxims to a concept used with considerable success to account for the features of semantic-pragmatic speech disorder described in Chapter 3, as well as many non-linguistic features of autism and Asperger's syndrome. This was a deficit in mentalising, metarepresentation or, as it is now universally known, theory of mind – the ability to construct a model of the mental states of other people.

Such an impairment could certainly lead to a failure to guide one's discourse according to the needs of the listener and so make speech difficult to follow. In Frith's (1992) hands the theory also had scope for explaining other schizophrenic symptoms. Unlike patients with autism and Asperger's syndrome, who fail to develop the ability to make inferences about the mental states of others, in schizophrenia there would likely be a breakdown in an ability the patients once had. This would cause them to continue to try and make inferences but to find the process difficult and produce ones that were faulty. They might then falsely infer that people were communicating with them when they were not, a plausible result of which could be delusions of reference and misinterpretation. Unable to read people's intentions properly, they might come to believe that people were deliberately disguising their intentions, and this could lead on to persecutory beliefs, which they would not then be able to easily dispel or correct through further observation. Failure to be aware of and attend to the mental states of others could plausibly also lead to impaired social interactions, and so result in the appearance of negative symptoms.[8]

Frith and later others went on to investigate the theory of mind in schizophrenia in a variety of ingenious ways. One of these was by means of the standard task used to demonstrate theory of mind deficit in autistic children, the false belief task, adapted for use in adults. Such tasks test whether one can understand a character in a story's false belief about the world (first-order false belief), and one character's false belief about another character's belief (second-order false belief). Frith and Corcoran (1996), Brüne (2003), Mazza *et al.* (2001) and Pickup and Frith (2001) all found evidence of impairment in schizophrenic patients on such tasks. Other studies had similar results using tasks assessing the ability of schizophrenic patients to understand the meaning behind hints, metaphor and irony

---

[8] In fact Frith's theory is broader still, as he proposes that patients with schizophrenia also have a lack of awareness of their *own* mental states, which he has linked theoretically to symptoms including auditory hallucinations, thought insertion and delusions of alien control.

(Corcoran *et al.*, 1995; Drury *et al.*, 1998; Langdon *et al.*, 2002), and the ability to appreciate humour understanding the mental states of the characters to get the joke (Corcoran *et al.*, 1997). Two studies (Corcoran and Frith, 1996; Tenyi *et al.*, 2002) even used a test of Gricean maxims. Some of these tests are summarised in Box 5.2.

Box 5.2 Some theory of mind tests used in schizophrenia

The hinting task (Corcoran *et al.*, 1995)
This tests the subject's ability to infer the real intentions behind indirect speech utterances. The task comprises ten short passages presenting an interaction between two characters. All of these end with one of the characters dropping a very obvious hint. The subjects were asked what the character really meant when he/she said this. If the subjects failed to give a correct response, more was added to the story in the shape of an even more obvious hint. The subjects were then asked what the character wants the other one to do.

Example:
Paul has to go to an interview and he's running late. While he's cleaning his shoes he says to his wife, Jane: 'I want to wear that blue shirt, but it's very creased.'

Question: What does Paul really mean when he says this?
Extra information: Paul goes on to say: 'It's in the ironing basket.'
Question: What does Paul want Jane to do?

Appreciation of visual jokes (Corcoran *et al.*, 1997)
Two sets of ten jokes were selected by the authors from magazines. The jokes in one set involved slapstick humour and could be understood in physical/behavioural terms. The jokes in the second set required an analysis of the main character's mental state. Seven out of the ten jokes depicted situations of false belief, where the main character believed something that onlookers knew not to be true. The three remaining jokes presented situations of deception, where one of the characters attempted to create a false belief in another character.

First-order false belief assessment: Object transfer task (used by Pickup and Frith, 2001)
This type of task assesses the ability to make an inference about a false belief about the state of the world. In the object transfer task, the subject must recognise that a story character has a false belief about the location of an object. The subject was shown a card depicting an office, common room and dining room in a

Box 5.2 (cont.)

hospital. A toy character (Andrew), who was a patient in the hospital, was introduced. The following story was then read aloud and enacted:

Andrew is in the common room, and has a book with him. Now he is going for lunch into the dining room and has left his book in the common room. While Andrew is away the nurse comes into the common room, picks up the book, and puts it into her office for safe-keeping.

ToM question: Where does Andrew think his book is?

Second-order false belief assessment: Burglar story (used by Mazza *et al.*, 2001 and Brüne, 2003).

Second-order false belief tasks assess the ability to understand a false belief about the belief of another character. Subjects were read the following story: A burglar has just robbed a bank and is running away from the police when he meets his brother. The burglar asks his brother not to let the police find him, then he runs away and hides in the church yard. The police have looked everywhere for the burglar except the church yard and the park. When they come across the burglar's brother they ask him if the burglar is in the church yard or in the park. They expect him to lie and so, wherever he tells them, they will go and look in the other place. But the Burglar's brother who is very clever and does want to save his brother knows that the police don't trust him.

ToM question: 'Where will the burglar's brother tell the police to look for the burglar. In the church yard or in the park?'
Control question: 'Where is the burglar really hiding?'

Grice's maxims (Tenyi *et al.*, 2002)

Four 'question and answer' vignettes were used, in which the maxim of relevance was violated to implicate a hidden, negative opinion behind the speaker's explicit utterance. Subjects were asked to judge these utterances and were evaluated by the investigators on a score from 1 to 2 points.

Vignette 1: a boss at a workplace is asked to give his opinion about his co-workers. About X, he says: 'I don't have any opinion about him.'
Vignette 2: a professor is asked to give his opinion about his junior lecturer. The answer is: 'She is a female.'
Vignette 3: students are asked about their teachers. A student says about teacher A: 'He is very young.'
Vignette 4: a teacher of art is asked about his students' talents. His answer about student B is: 'She has an attractive body.'

As a theory of schizophrenic symptoms, theory of mind deficit needs to clear the hurdle that it is not just part of the pattern of general intellectual impairment associated with the disorder which, as discussed in Chapter 4, would tend to show itself as poor performance on any test. In general, Frith and co-workers have been quite scrupulous about addressing this issue, by, for example, showing that significant impairment on false belief tests remained when subgroups of patients and controls matched for current IQ were compared (e.g. Corcoran *et al.*, 1995; 1997; Frith and Corcoran, 1996; Pickup and Frith, 2001). Most other studies have also found that theory of mind impairment survives controlling for general intellectual impairment (Mazza *et al.*, 2001; Langdon *et al.*, 2002). Only one study (Brüne *et al.*, 2003) found that matching for current IQ attenuated the differences between schizophrenic patients and controls to the point of non-significance.

The other important challenge is to establish that theory of mind impairment is associated with the schizophrenic symptoms it purports to explain, including thought disorder. Almost all studies have addressed this, though sometimes in complicated and not particularly transparent ways. This applies particularly to the studies of Frith's group, which have adopted a strategy of isolating groups of patients who only show a single class of symptom – negative symptoms, persecutory and/or referential delusions, passivity experiences, and so on – and testing them for the presence or absence of deficit in accordance with the predictions of the theory. Nevertheless, even in these studies it is possible to extract correlations between impairment on theory of mind tasks and positive, negative and disorganisation symptoms. These and the correlations from other studies are shown in Table 5.5. It is evident that the studies consistently found associations with negative symptoms. Several also found significant or near significant associations with positive symptoms (delusions and hallucinations). However, only a minority of studies found significant correlations with the disorganisation syndrome.

Conclusion

A dysfunction at the level of communicative competence has strong intuitive appeal as an explanation for the difficult-to-follow quality of thought-disordered speech. But at the same time communicative competence is a broad term, which covers a number of quite different areas of language use. There is no particular reason to expect all of these to be implicated in thought disorder, and this is what the fairly limited evidence to date tends to suggest.

There is definite support for an abnormality in discourse knowledge, or at least one aspect of this. The numbers of relevant studies are small and their sample sizes are often not much larger, but almost without fail they have found that patients with thought disorder use referential ties in an unclear, ambiguous or even frankly

Table 5.5 Correlations between impairment on different theory of mind tasks and schizophrenic syndromes

	Positive symptoms	Disorganisation/ thought disorder	Negative symptoms
1st-order false belief	✗[5] ✗[8]	✗[5] ✗[8]	✓[5] ✗[8]
2nd-order false belief	✗[5] ✗[8]	✗[5] ✗[8]	✓[3] ✗[5] ✗[8]
False belief	✗[6] ✓/✗[7]	✗[7]	✓[6] ✓[7]
Inferring intentions		✓[4]	
Comprehension of metaphor	✗[7]	✗[7]	✓[7]
Comprehension of irony	✓[7]	✓[7]	✗[7]
Hinting task	✓/✗[2]		✓[2]
Politeness/tactfulness	✓/✗[1]		✓[1]
Gricean Maxims	✗[1]		✓[1]

Notes: ✓/✗ – Significant at trend level.
[1]Corcoran and Frith (1996)
[2]Corcoran *et al.* (1995)
[3]Doody *et al.* (1998)
[4]Sarfati *et al.* (1999a, b)
[5]Mazza *et al.* (2001)
[6]Pickup and Frith (2001)
[7]Langdon *et al.* (2002)
[8]Pollice *et al.* (2002)

erroneous way. This may or may not be superimposed on a general reduction in use of cohesive ties in schizophrenia as a whole. The fact that it is semantic ties which appear to be affected is an unexpected bonus for the theme of semantic abnormality that emerged in the last chapter and will be developed further in the next.

There are suggestions that thought-disordered patients do not take context into account when listening to speech. But with the evidence base standing at essentially two studies, there is not much scope for stronger conclusions. Another limitation is that both Chapman and Chapman (1973) and Kuperberg *et al.* (1998) had to rely on argument rather than experiment in order to make the case that what they found would also lead to a failure to take context into account when speaking.

The studies reviewed in this chapter indicate compellingly that impaired theory of mind is one of the few cognitive deficits in schizophrenia which is primarily associated with symptoms rather than with general intellectual impairment. In the shape of a failure to pay attention to the listener's needs, this theory also has formidable power to explain thought disorder. But the evidence is simply not there. Thought-disordered schizophrenic patients do not appear to have a pragmatic impairment in the same way that people with autism and Asperger syndrome do.

6

Thought disorder as a dysexecutive phenomenon

Just over twenty years ago, Schwartz (1982) critically reviewed a number of cognitive psychological approaches to thought disorder in existence at the time. He found most of them wanting, by virtue of what he considered to be errors in their experimental methods, faulty observations, tautological reasoning or theoretical models that were too simple. The targets of his attack included virtually all the leading theories of the day, such as Goldstein's (1944) impairment of abstract thinking (not found in studies using properly matched controls), Von Domarus' (1944) failure to adhere to the laws of normal logic (unsupported by actual studies of reasoning in schizophrenic patients), Chapman and Chapman's (1973) bias to the strong meaning of words (not specific to thought disorder) and Salzinger *et al.*'s (1978) so-called immediacy hypothesis, which proposed that verbal behaviour was excessively controlled by stimuli in the environment (better explained in other terms).

One of the few cognitive approaches which escaped Schwartz's criticism was overinclusive thinking, discussed in the next chapter. Another he remained optimistic about was a disorder of attention; this was not the then fashionable theory that schizophrenic patients were unable to filter out unwanted information from consciousness (which Schwartz disapproved of on theoretical grounds and was not destined to stand the test of time), but a more active form of attention concerned with the selection of responses. By this point Schwartz – and others including Harrow, Chaika and Frith as described below – were closing in on a novel account of thought disorder, as a failure in what was just beginning to be called executive function, the high-level strategic control of behaviour, specifically speech behaviour.

However, the term executive function was being introduced to replace the older term frontal lobe function, and so this new theory was essentially neuro-psychological rather than cognitive psychological in orientation. While this was welcome in the fledgling DSM III era, and converged with a number of findings that were emerging from other areas of biological schizophrenia research, it did mean constructing an account which could move from a neurological syndrome associated with damage to the frontal lobes, to a symptom of a psychiatric disorder which on the face of it was very different, via a cognitive function which was not very well understood. This was never going to be a straightforward exercise, and in this chapter each step of the argument is considered separately.

The frontal lobe syndrome

The symptoms and signs seen after damage to the frontal lobes, or more precisely the prefrontal cortex and its subcortical connections, seem at first sight a long way from attention and the strategic control of behaviour. The most immediately obvious features of the syndrome are in the realm of personality and behaviour, where they take the form of apathy, unconcern, impulsiveness, irresponsibility and disinhibition. These can occur in different combinations in different patients or sometimes in the same patient at different times. Sometimes the picture is predominantly one of apathy. For example, Blumer and Benson (1975) described a patient who had previously been outgoing and active, but, after sustaining frontal lobe damage in a road traffic accident, spent most of his time sitting alone smoking; he never initiated a conversation or made a request, and showed a complete lack of interest in his wife and children. In other cases, though, the changes are in the reverse direction and the patient becomes restless, active and interfering. Thus, another of Blumer and Benson's patients was outspoken, facetious, brash and disrespectful and much given to making morbid jokes. Many patients of both types of presentation are tactless and irresponsible and show socially and sexually disinhibited behaviour. Heinrichs (2001) described one patient who nearly lost his job as a teacher after he started making sexual comments to his students in class, and another who wrote a sexually explicit letter to his therapist, suggesting they run away together, and was amused and bewildered at the reaction of his family when they found out.

The cognitive changes that patients with the frontal lobe syndrome show are at least as difficult to try and make sense of. While intelligence can remain normal or show only a slight decline, the patients have difficulty grasping complicated problems and are unable to master novel tasks. However, they may be well able to work along routine lines, prompting the observation that they can often perform surprisingly well, provided that there is someone else to act as their frontal lobes for them (Baddeley and Wilson, 1986). Another paradox is that the patients may be distractible and unable to concentrate on any task for more than a few moments, but at the same time can be remarkably fixed and repetitive in speech and behaviour.

On neuropsychological testing frontal lobe patients show impairment on tasks requiring them to develop and use strategies in a flexible way. The prototypical test of this type is the Wisconsin Card Sorting Test in which the subject has to sort cards according to rules which he or she has to work out by trial and error and which change unpredictably from time to time. The patients learn the initial sorting principle without difficulty, but continue to sort the cards according to this rule when it changes, and thus make many perseverative errors. Beyond this, there is impairment on a wide range of tasks which have few obvious features in common, apart from the fact that they seem to require strategy, decision making and checking. A case which illustrates the frontal pattern of cognitive impairment and which also gives a graphic account of the syndrome, including some of its lesser-known features, is described in Box 6.1.

Box 6.1 RJ: a patient with the dysexecutive syndrome due to bilateral frontal lobe damage

(From Baddeley, 1986; Baddeley and Wilson, 1986; 1988; Baddeley, 1990)

The patient suffered a serious head injury when his car ran into the back of a horsebox. He was unconscious for several weeks, but gradually recovered physically. A CT scan showed haemorrhages in both frontal lobes.

After the accident, his behaviour ranged from being passive and apathetic (e.g. on occasions he sat in the same chair without speaking or moving for two hours) to being amusing and charming. He perseverated in speech, writing and other motor responses. For example, when asked to write the meaning of 'Too many cooks spoil the broth' he wrote 'too many skills . . . for such a mess of of of of of of a mess of of . . .' and so on. Instructed to measure out a piece of string in order to cut it later, he immediately started to cut and when told not to, replied 'Yes I know I'm not to cut it', meanwhile continuing to cut. He had great difficulty in planning his activities or in combining separate pieces of information. His reasoning skills were also impaired. He was totally unable to answer questions such as 'There were 18 books on two shelves. Twice as many books were on one shelf as the other. How many books were on each shelf?' He was however not at all dysphasic.

RJ was a trained engineer and had an estimated premorbid IQ in the region of 120. When tested several months after his accident, his verbal IQ was in the region of 100, while his performance IQ had dropped to 76. On the modified Wisconsin Card Sorting Test he was able to achieve no categories, making a total of forty-five errors of which forty-three were perseverations. His performance on the Cognitive Estimates Test, which requires the subject to answer questions such as: *How fast do racehorses gallop?* and *What is the age of the oldest person alive in Britain today?*, gave a raw score of 8, again indicating frontal lobe damage. Another indication of the classic pattern was an impairment in verbal fluency. When required to generate as many words as possible beginning with S and V he failed to generate any item in the 90 seconds available, commenting, 'There must be hundreds of them!' When asked to generate animals he generated only one.

Box 6.1 (cont.)

While his digit span was within the normal range, his long-term learning ability was very substantially impaired. His performance on the Wechsler Logical Memory Test was extremely poor on both immediate and delayed tests. He also showed impaired performance in copying and gross impairment in recalling the Rey figure, a result that probably reflected a combination of perceptual, memory and planning problems. In learning novel tasks, his lack of flexibility and tendency to stereotyped behaviour was a major problem.

RJ could not remember his past reliably and confabulation was a marked feature of his behaviour. When asked about his accident he would always volunteer a detailed description. On each occasion the description was different, the only common feature being that he was involved in a car crash and that he remained conscious throughout. In actual fact he was unconscious for several weeks following the accident. This tendency to confabulate was tested by giving him certain cue words and asking him if they reminded him of a particular incident that he himself had experienced. This produced a number of rather colourful incidents, which were delivered with the appearance of complete conviction, with full environmental detail. For example the cue word 'river' evoked an 'incident' where he had taken his niece rowing on the river, had subsequently got out of the boat, called to her and, when she turned, thrown a stone that hit her eye. This was followed by an elaborate description of taking her to hospital, a word-by-word account of his conversation with the doctor and so forth. When subsequently given the same cue he produced a completely different recall and denied any knowledge of the previous incident, an incident which his wife confirmed had not occurred.

In addition to confabulating incidents that had not occurred he also denied all knowledge of events that had. For example, on one occasion while spending the weekend at home from the rehabilitation centre, he turned to his wife in bed and asked her:

Why do you keep telling people we are married?

But we are married; we have two children.

That doesn't mean that we are married!

At this point his wife got out of bed and produced their wedding photographs. RJ looked at them carefully then replied:

That chap certainly looks like me, but it's not me!

The dysexecutive syndrome

Baddeley (1986) proposed this term to try and capture the elusive pattern of cognitive deficits seen in patients with frontal lobe lesions. He based his account on a model of a 'supervisory attentional system' developed earlier by Norman and

Shallice (1980; Shallice, 1982). This model assumes that behaviour is controlled at two levels. Schemas for routine behaviours are triggered and run off in response to the appropriate perceptual stimuli, and the conflicts that arise between them from time to time are resolved by an automatic system of 'contention scheduling'. The supervisory attentional system, as its name suggests, is called into play to override these automatically triggered routine behaviours in circumstances where conscious decisions are required. These circumstances include novelty, danger, situations where planning or decision-making is necessary, and those where a strong habitual response has to be inhibited.

Although typically seen in association with damage to the frontal lobes, for a number of reasons Baddeley considered it desirable to specify the dysexecutive syndrome purely as a particular form of cognitive deficit. One reason for this was the limited power of the model to account for the changes in personality and behaviour described above. In fact, many patients have been described in whom there is a dissociation between impairment on frontal tests and behaviour. It also reflected an important principle in neuropsychology, particularly British neuropsychology, of separating a cognitive dysfunction from its alleged anatomical substrate. As Baddeley (1996) put it:

> The model is principally a functional model that would exist and be useful even if there proved to be no simple mapping on to underlying neuroanatomy. To add a component that was defined neuroanatomically rather than functionally would therefore be anomalous. It would also be likely to be unhelpful, bearing in mind the fact that the frontal lobes constitute an extremely large area that almost certainly has multiple functions that are as yet poorly understood. It is entirely possible that, although the frontal lobes are often involved in many executive processes, other parts of the brain may also be involved in executive control. If we identify the central executive exclusively with frontal function, then we might well find ourselves excluding from the central executive processes that are clearly executive in nature, simply because they prove not to be frontally located. Equally, we would be in danger of describing functions as executive simply because they were based on the frontal lobes.

This distinction, and the way it has sometimes failed to be appreciated, forms an important counterpoint to the development of thinking about frontal lobe and executive dysfunction in thought disorder.

Schizophrenia and the frontal lobes

Nowadays the concept of frontal dysfunction is so firmly entrenched in psychiatric thinking, and so uncritically invoked to account for many diverse features of schizophrenia and other disorders, that David (1992) felt obliged to write a paper with the title: 'Frontal lobology: psychiatry's new pseudoscience'. Yet this was not always the case. Although it is often implied that speculation about the role of the frontal lobes in schizophrenia stretches back in an unbroken tradition to Kraepelin (1913a), he in fact he only referred to them as a possible site of pathology in passing, along with the temporal lobes and the sensorimotor cortex. Until comparatively recently the only other author who advocated a frontal lobe theory of schizophrenia was Kleist (e.g. 1960), thereby almost guaranteeing its continued obscurity.

What changed the frontal lobes from a region of no particular interest in schizophrenia to a powerful force driving research was the introduction of functional brain imaging. In the first study to use this technique, Ingvar and Franzen (1974) found that chronic schizophrenic patients showed a loss of the normal pattern of greater regional blood flow[1] in anterior as opposed to posterior regions, a pattern they referred to as 'hypofrontality'. This was followed by many further studies, some but not all of which confirmed the finding. Somewhat later Weinberger *et al.* (1986) started a second wave of studies when they argued that hypofrontality might be more reliably demonstrated by carrying out functional imaging while schizophrenic patients were engaged in tasks that made demands on the frontal lobes. They found that a group of chronic schizophrenic patients showed only a trend to hypofrontality at rest, but markedly failed to activate the prefrontal cortex when they performed the Wisconsin Card Sorting Test. This too was followed by a stream of further studies, which has continued unabated to the present day.

The finding of hypofrontality also launched a generation of structural imaging studies. With one abnormality, lateral ventricular enlargement, already documented in schizophrenia (see Chapter 2), a number of studies also found evidence that the frontal lobes were smaller than normal. There were also claims from a steady trickle of post-mortem brain studies that a variety of histological abnormalities could be demonstrated in the prefrontal cortex of schizophrenic patients.

All this obscured the fact that hypofrontality has never been a well-replicated finding in schizophrenia. Reviewing the field in 1995, Chua and McKenna found that hypofrontality was present at rest in only ten of twenty-seven studies which employed respectable numbers of patients and controls. Activation hypofrontality, where positive and negative findings were approximately equally divided, fared only slightly better.

What rescues hypofrontality from a verdict of non-replication is meta-analysis. Two such studies (Davidson and Heinrichs, 2003; Hill *et al.*, 2004), reviewing somewhat different sets of findings, found overall support for the reality of the finding, under both resting and activation conditions. One of these is summarised in Box 6.2. However, the same cannot be said for structural brain abnormality.

---

[1] Regional blood flow changes with changes in regional metabolism, and so is often used as an index of brain activity.

A meta-analysis of MRI studies by Wright *et al.* (2000) has made it clear that any frontal lobe volume reductions in schizophrenia are no greater than those of around 3% found for the brain as a whole. This is also summarised in Box 6.2. As for neuropathological studies, these sail on as one of the least reputable areas of biological schizophrenia research, oblivious to criticisms about their small sample sizes, failure to use appropriate controls and the complete lack of consistent findings from study to study.

Box 6.2 Structural and functional frontal lobe abnormality in schizophrenia: two meta-analyses

Structural brain abnormality
In contrast to an earlier generation of CT scan studies, many of which used control groups which were likely to have overestimated the differences in schizophrenia, MRI studies have typically compared patients to well-matched prospectively ascertained volunteers.

Wright *et al.* (2000) meta-analysed 58 MRI studies comparing schizophrenic patients to normal controls. This revealed a substantial increase in lateral ventricular volume, of the order of 20–30%. Brain volume, however, was 97–99% of that in normal subjects. The corresponding figures for frontal lobe volume were 92–98% (left) and 93–97% (right). These decreases were not clearly disproportionate to the reduction in whole brain volume. Larger reductions were found for the medial temporal lobe structures of the amygdala and parahippocampal gyrus.

Brain structure	No. of studies	Total N	Effect size (d)	% of normal volume in schizophrenia
Left lateral ventricle	18	1053	0.51	130
Right lateral ventricle	18	1053	0.39	120
Whole brain	31	1867	−0.25	98
Left frontal lobe	13	762	−0.34	95
Right frontal lobe	13	762	−0.36	95

Functional brain abnormality
Functional imaging studies in schizophrenia have used a range of imaging techniques, including [133]Xenon, SPECT and PET, and have measured hypofrontality in a variety of different ways. An important difference of the latter type concerns use of 'absolute' measures of frontal blood flow/metabolism in contrast to 'relative' measures, which correct for whole brain blood flow/metabolism. Hypofrontality has been also examined at rest and also under conditions of neuropsychological task activation.

Box 6.2 (cont.)

Hill *et al.* (2004) meta-analysed studies comparing schizophrenic patients and normal controls at rest and under activation conditions. Hypofrontality was supported in both, with the effect size falling into the small to medium range.

	No. of studies	Total N	Effect size (d)	Approx. degree of non-overlap (%)
Whole brain	22	795	−0.26 (−0.40/−0.11)	20
Resting hypofrontality (relative)	38	1474	−0.32 (−0.43/−0.21)	25
Resting hypofrontality (absolute)	25	950	−0.55 (−0.68/−0.41)	33
Activation hypofrontality (relative)	17	685	−0.37 (−0.53/−0.22)	25
Activation hypofrontality (absolute)	10	347	−0.42 (−0.65/−0.20)	30

Neuroleptic treatment appeared to be responsible for at least some of a small reduction in whole brain blood flow/metabolism in schizophrenia, but this factor did not account for hypofrontality. Values for hypofrontality did not vary significantly across the different techniques used. An unexpected finding was an apparent association with chronicity of illness. Studies examining first episode patients or those with a mean duration of less than two years showed no hypofrontality, whereas those carried out on mixed or purely chronic patient groups showed progressively more evidence of this.

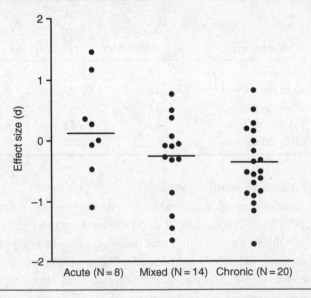

So is there a dysexecutive syndrome in schizophrenia?

Neuropsychological studies of executive function only began to be undertaken late in the course of the frontal initiative in schizophrenia research, almost as it were as an afterthought. The first studies were carried out by Weinberger and co-workers (Goldberg et al., 1987, 1988) in the wake of their study of activation hypofrontality, and these and several other studies which followed were unanimous in finding impairment on a range of executive tasks. By and large, these studies managed to ignore the possibility, discussed in Chapter 4, that what was being held up as evidence of a specific dysexecutive syndrome in schizophrenia was merely a part of the overall intellectual impairment seen in the disorder, which would show itself on any test. When Laws (1999) reviewed thirty-three studies using the Wisconsin Card Sorting Test he found that half failed to include any non-executive measures for comparison purposes, and almost all of the remainder failed to find any evidence that executive function was selectively impaired.

Establishing that a deficit is specific against a background of varying degrees of general intellectual impairment is not easy and there is no universally agreed method for doing so, let alone one that is foolproof. A few studies have documented impairment on executive tests in schizophrenic patients selected for meeting some standard of overall intellectual intactness (e.g. Elliott et al., 1995, 1998; Evans et al., 1997). Others have attempted to covary out the effects of IQ (e.g. Crawford et al., 1993). But probably the most convincing demonstration is in the single case study of Shallice et al. (1991) described in Chapter 4. All five of the chronically hospitalised schizophrenic patients in this study showed multiple failures on tests sensitive to frontal lobe dysfunction, including the two patients with preserved general intellectual function, HE and HS, who failed three and four of the ten tests respectively (see Chapter 4, Table 4.2). These two patients showed no corresponding failures on the tests of visual, visuospatial function and language, although they did show scattered failures on the memory tests in the battery.

Ultimately, though, it may not matter whether or not executive impairment in schizophrenia is a specific neuropsychological deficit in the sense of being disproportionate to the overall level of intellectual impairment. In a commentary on Laws' (1999) review, Frith (1999) wrote.

First, not all patients with schizophrenia perform badly on frontal lobe tests. Second, in those patients that do perform badly there is usually evidence of a more general intellectual impairment. Third, poor performance on tests of executive function does not necessarily mean executive impairments or frontal lobe damage. All sensible and informed people would agree with these points . . . I would suggest that we should not expect to find a characteristic neuropsychology associated with schizophrenia. Schizophrenia is a diagnostic category including patients who show a wide range of signs and symptoms which fluctuate over time. Although it is still possible that there is a specific biological marker associated with this disease I do not think that we should expect to find a specific psychological marker. In contrast, it is reasonable to expect to find psychological markers for particular signs and symptoms.

One of the symptoms which Frith had in mind when he wrote this was thought disorder.

Thought disorder as frontal/executive dysfunction

In the years following Schwartz's (1982) review several prototypes for a dysexecutive theory of thought disorder appeared. As described in Chapter 1, Harrow and co-workers' rediscovery of the phenomenon of interpenetration of themes led them to suggest that a factor underlying it might be a failure in 'specific aspects of the executive function . . . involved in controlling and guiding language and behavior' (Harrow and Prosen, 1978; see also Harrow and Miller, 1980; Harrow et al., 1983). At around the same time Chaika (1982) proposed a unifying account of the errors she identified in thought-disordered speech, based on 'two underlying dysfunctions: inappropriate perseverations combined with lack of control over the selection of linguistic material'. Frith (1987) was also moving towards the general theory of schizophrenia outlined in Chapter 5, in which his hypothesised failure to take into account listeners' needs reflected abnormality at 'the highest levels of language processing, involved in the planning and execution of discourse' (Frith, 1992).

It was, however, McGrath (1991) who assembled these ideas into a systematic theory, which could relate the diverse elements of thought disorder to symptoms associated with the frontal lobe syndrome and/or the dysexecutive syndrome. The main points of his argument were as follows:

Failure to establish a set: Lack of a general intention to talk could obviously result in the symptom of poverty of speech. In fact, as McGrath pointed out, something seemingly identical to this symptom is seen in frontal lobe patients, where it is part of, or shades into, the general picture of apathy. Initiation of speech also requires generation of a topic focus to guide the communication. Failure to establish a proper topic set could lead to the patient conveying little information, and so give rise to poverty of content of speech.

Inability to change set: Perseveration was included as a feature of thought disorder by Andreasen (1979a), and this is also one of the classic features of the dysexecutive syndrome. McGrath also argued that the concept of perseveration could be extended to account for some of the other abnormalities seen in thought disorder. Clang associations could be understood as perseveration of the phonological features of words at the expense of their meaning. Perseveration of phrases and sentences would lead to repetitiveness of speech, one of the factors Andreasen (1979a) identified as contributing to poverty of content of speech. Perseveration of theme, coupled with a failure to suppress a bizarre delusion or intrusive thought, could provide a basis for interpenetration of themes.

Failure of planning and editing: When a speaker only has to make a short statement, respond to simple questions or relate an incident chronologically, he or she can draw on in-built templates and stock patterns of discourse. For anything more complicated, however, he or she must plan a linear sequence of communication out of an almost infinite variety of possible combinations and permutations of the relevant ideas. Failure to do so would place an excessive burden on the listener, and incidentally violate most of Grice's conversational maxims.

Failure to monitor errors: In addition to planning and editing of speech, constant checking is also required to ensure that the listener is comprehending what is being said. If such monitoring were not carried out, the speaker would fail to notice when the listener was becoming confused by virtue of one or more of the above abnormalities and so compound the above problems.

McGrath (1991) concluded his account by proposing two testable hypotheses. One of these was the straightforward prediction that thought-disordered patients should show impairment on some but not all tests of executive function, specifically those measuring the ability to establish, maintain and change sets, and those designed to measure planning. The other was that thought disorder should not be restricted to schizophrenia and mania, but should be observable in any disorder where there is frontal lobe dysfunction, where it should be associated with the same pattern of impairment on executive tests. The first of these proposals has been extensively put to the test and is discussed in a later section. The second has not been taken up to any extent, but the core of McGrath's prediction is that patients with frontal lobe lesions should sometimes show thought disorder. It should be possible to decide this by consulting the neurological literature.

Speech in patients with the frontal lobe syndrome

Unfortunately, the literature on speech in patients with frontal lobe lesions is anything but rich. Most descriptions of the frontal lobe syndrome either fail to mention speech at all, or merely rehearse the standard view that it is laconic, simple, repetitive and concrete. Nevertheless, here and there allusions to more interesting phenomena can be found, such as: 'A tendency exists toward perseveration, confabulation and free association of ideas' (Novoa and Ardila, 1987);

'Social appropriateness, narrative coherence, and veracity may be most severely damaged'; and 'Tangential, irrelevant comments are frequent and a vague rambling quality characterizes their verbal communication' (both from Alexander et al., 1989).

Blumer and Benson (1975) went further, drawing attention to the distinction, alluded to above, between two forms of the frontal lobe syndrome. One was an apathetic or a 'pseudodepressed' type characterised by inactivity, slowness and indifference, and the other was a disinhibited or 'pseudopsychopathic' type in which the patient showed a lack of normal tact and restraint and was prone to impulsive behaviour and outbursts of anger. Describing a case of the latter type, Blumer and Benson stated that the patient was not aphasic but misused words in a manner that suggested inability to maintain specific meanings. In answer to a question about whether the injury had affected his thinking, for example, he replied: 'Yeah – it's affected the way I think – it's affected my senses – the only things I can taste are sugar and salt – I can't detect a pungent odor – ha ha – to tell you the truth it's a blessing this way.' When the question was repeated his response was, 'Yes – I'm not as spry on my feet as I was before.'

Kaczmarek (1984) formally investigated speech in a study of patients with brain tumours in different locations. His sample included forty-five patients with frontal lobe tumours, made up of fifteen with a left dorsolateral localisation, fifteen with a left orbitofrontal localisation and fifteen in whom the lesion was right-sided, plus groups of fifteen patients with posterior tumours with or without aphasia; there were also fifteen normal controls. All the subjects were engaged in a range of tasks, such as repeating stories and describing pictures, as well as talking on various topics. The findings are shown in Table 6.1. As a group the frontal lobe patients produced only slightly more perseverative responses than the other groups. However, the rate was twice as high in the subgroup of patients with left dorsolateral lesions. Confabulations were also higher in the frontal patients compared with the remaining patients, and use of stereotyped phrases were only seen in this group. What Kaczmarek called digressions were seen almost exclusively in the frontal patients, where they were most pronounced in those with left orbitofrontal lesions, the area traditionally associated with the disinhibited form of the frontal lobe syndrome. This group also showed a high rate of misnamings.

Another neurological disorder that presents with the frontal lobe syndrome is fronto-temporal dementia (Gustafson, 1987; Hodges, 1993; Snowden et al., 1996).[2] Patients with the frontal variant of this disease develop typical frontal personality changes, sometimes with additional features such as complex

---

[2] This is similar to and replaces the older term Pick's disease. However, it is a broader concept, principally because only about half of patients show the typical histological changes of Pick's disease at post-mortem.

Table 6.1 Proportion of different kinds of abnormality in the speech of patients with frontal and non-frontal lesions (% of total utterances)

(From Kaczmarek, 1984, reprinted with permission from Elsevier)

	Frontal	Posterior with aphasia	Posterior without aphasia	Controls
Perseveration	29.0[1]	24.4	22.2	22.3
Confabulation	27.7	8.9	4.2	6.5
Stereotyped phrases	17.3	–	–	–
Misnamings	13.0[2]	38.5	10.6	3.3
Digressions	10.2	1.3	–	–
Mispronunciations	–	25.6	–	–
Correct utterances	2.8	1.3	63.9	67.9

Notes: [1]Patients with left dorsolateral frontal lesions showed 56.0% perseverations, compared with 21.2% in those with left orbitofrontal lesions and 9.6% in those with right frontal lesions.
[2]Patients with left orbitofrontal lesions showed 25.6% misnamings, compared with 5.0% in those with left dorsolateral lesions and 8.5% in those with right frontal lesions.

stereotyped behaviour and compulsive eating, before ultimately progressing to a state of severe akinesia and mutism. As in the frontal lobe syndrome due to head injury, strokes, tumours and so on, the clinical picture may take apathetic and disinhibited forms. In one of the studies which established the existence of the disorder, Neary *et al.* (1988) described two patients with the latter presentation. One showed 'a press of speech, which was frequently off the point, and contained stereotyped phrases and play-on-words, which amused her'. There was some word-finding difficulty, and she made occasional verbal paraphasic errors, although there was no disorder of syntax. The other patient was similar in that his speech was rapid and frequently off the point; he would also spontaneously break into song, or relate rhymes, and he produced puns and stereotyped phrases. However, he did not show paraphasias.

But for a really detailed account of speech in the frontal lobe syndrome, one has to turn to the psychiatric literature on frontal lobotomy or leucotomy. A large proportion of the patients who were subjected to this procedure are not a useful source of evidence, since they were suffering from schizophrenia – a disorder which, in the words of Gray and McNaughton (2000), many thousands of gratuitous operations later it was found to be absolutely no use for. Even in the next largest group of patients operated on, those with depression, there could still be dispute over how much any changes in speech were due to the pre-existing mental disorder. However, there have always been a small number of patients who have undergone leucotomy for intractable neurotic disorders. Two studies examined groups of such patients before and after surgery, with the specific aim of identifying the effects of removal of the prefrontal cortex on personality. Their studies also provide valuable data on its effects on language and thought.

Petrie (1952) collected data from a series of twenty patients who underwent prefrontal leucotomy mainly for obsessional neurosis and anxiety states; some had a diagnosis of depression without psychotic symptoms and one or two had hysterical symptoms. Before surgery, he gave the patients a range of cognitive tests, which included interpreting proverbs and defining words. When these were re-administered three and nine months after operation, they revealed changes in the patients' use of language which went beyond the familiar concreteness, perseveration and loss of richness of thought. For example, when interpreting proverbs, some patients showed a tendency to jump from one idea to another 'far less relevant though in some way associated with the original idea'. When giving definitions, common words were misused and answers were given which only approximated to the patients' intended meaning. Thus one patient defined a fable as 'a far-reaching tale'; another said a nail was 'a metal joiner', a spade was 'a utensil for gardening' and a sword was 'an article for killing animals'. Another patient said that fur could be used 'as a wearing apparatus'.

Some patients also showed an increase in the use of exclamations, rhetorical questions and sweeping general statements, which imparted a bombastic style to their speech and writing. For example, one patient interpreted *Never judge a book by its cover* as, 'Whether the outside be neat or otherwise, it is the internals which will suggest the wealth of the thing.' Another wrote in an essay: 'An unbearable temper is just another general incident which finally wraps up into your final countenance which to one and all is something to be admired.'

Tow (1955) described generally similar changes in a series of thirty-six patients with a variety of neurotic diagnoses, including anorexia nervosa and hypochondriasis (three were also stated to be paranoid and one had an additional diagnosis of epilepsy). Before the operation, he asked the patients to write an autobiography. There were no restrictions on the length or content of this, and they were asked to write as much as they could about their attitudes and feelings towards things, to include their likes and dislikes and to describe not only events but also their emotional reactions to them. A year later, they were then asked to write another account, this time of the events following the operation. Sometimes the effects of surgery were brutal. One patient who had given an articulate, insightful and quite long account of his life before the operation, wrote the following afterwards:

Upon general reserection first thing in the morning I used to generally partake in normale games in the wards, and used to after general amusement in the wards I used to have a game of billiards after dinner, and after general games I used to go out and do some work upon the farm.

In other cases, though, the changes were in a different direction. Along with a general scrappiness and uninformativeness, there was a tendency towards word play, artificiality, literariness and even pedantry. Tow quoted two patients, one of whose style became peculiar, eccentric and ruminative, with alliterations and occasional neologisms, and the other whose writing was essentially nonsensical. These are shown in Box 6.3. The points of similarity to schizophrenic thought disorder (and in the first case, it has to be said, to the writings of Joyce) are not easy to dismiss.

Box 6.3 Extracts from the written accounts of two patients before and a year after undergoing prefrontal leucotomy

(From Tow, 1955)

Subject 28

Before operation
At nine I went to Chartdean, where I was, to a certain extent, licked into shape. I grew too tough and tall to ever become a successful professional ballet dancer, so gave that up and zipped through my school career doing as little work as quickly and successfully as could be. At 14 I weighed nearly 11 stone, and was given a joke plunket roller as a birthday present! Furious, I decided to 'slim' and ate less. Mary was on the same tack, and we vied with each other to deny our healthy schoolgirl appetites.

At 17 I met Cedric, who instantly decided on me only, and has never seriously looked upon anyone else since. We trotted around London and did everything together, and the day before I went to Paris to 'finish', he asked me to marry him. I didn't seriously love him at all, but he was so earnest that I hadn't the strength to say so, and tried to hedge and went to France for six months, still slimming.

After operation
My feelings now cannot but be very closely allied with those previous to my operation, and forever with me but tinted by the certainty that they are not, and can never be parallel with them. For me, the feelings are always tainted by my questionings, 'Can these things be so, and if they are so, is it due to the loocotome?' (Poor spelling due to my ignorance.) And so on ad lib., until my own private handiwork-of-brain became a mere negative nonchalance behind the entire great

Box 6.3 (cont.)

loocotome-caused-get-at. Or so it seems to me now, though I do but readily realise that this is not forever so in every small event, and that I do indeed, frequently work forgetting the whole operation, its cause, cost and effect. How to retrace these I can hardly now imagine, though at one time there were vast reasons for them all. Now it is enough to retrace one's memories, their cause and effect . . . their cause and their result. You are so firm and so resolute and I stand here so wary and uncertain – so dallying in my ways and opinions.

At night all is dull despair and destitution: I lie in indigence and lack of strength. All my will is overcome with dull despair and diffidence: there is no force within me left to overcome fatigue and daydeadness. At night, if I can at last manage to climb into bed, I usually wet it two or three times . . . *which* annoys me very much. Everywhere on professional grounds I am assured that this will soon lessen into nothingness, but I myself regard this as the forming of an unbreaking habit. So what . . . ?

Subject 17

Before operation

My parents on both sides were of Scottish Ancestry being first cousins. My Mother's parents were Scots farmers living near Dumfries about five miles out in the Parish of Kirkmahoe. It is from them, I think, that I inherit my love of animals, country life and the out of doors, as although my mother came to London, living and working with a Court Dressmaker, she never loved town life as much as country life. One of our greatest joys was a visit to cousins in the same parish. Uncle being delicate, bred Highland cattle. Some of my happiest moments have been spent walking around farms, gathering eggs etc. being 'introduced' to goats, calves, new born lambs etc. and that beautiful joy of going around 'gathering eggs' warm from the nest.

After operation

I am beginning to long *very much* for a normal life – freedom from medical supervision of my mind (of which I do not approve!) and complete freedom of action and will – also a longing to cease from hearing of the complete worldly wisdom *'spiritual well being of the Matrons'* (*Especially* the Matron of the past *Matron B*) the beautity of one of the *Irish* Sisters whom every man in the Hospital *adores* her *small waist*, and *ample arm above*, *adored*, as I hear *especially* by Dr – , the *ravishing beauty* of *M.C.* her *unbounded cheek*, her *ravishing wits* (although she has been *'reported* to say "her brain is mine – and mine is hers!!" as according to what I hear she has been appointed by Padre to instruct me how to *live a Christian Life*

and obey Dr – 's orders to lie, cheat, steal thieve and break all the ten command-
ments, according to *Hospitals orders*!!! This of course I do not talk about, but only
think about (but some how feel my thoughts are read by electricity!) in case the
"Medical Staff" say I have delusions *which of course I have not*!!

Liddle and the neuropsychology of disorganisation

Even before McGrath developed the frontal/executive hypothesis of thought
disorder into a fully fledged theory, Liddle (1987b) had made a start on testing
its main prediction. He surmised that the positive, negative and disorganisation
syndromes he isolated in the factor-analytic study described in Chapter 2 were a
reflection of different underlying pathological processes, and might therefore be
associated with – perhaps even result from – different neuropsychological deficits.
He therefore administered a range of neuropsychological tests to the forty-seven
patients in his original study and correlated performance on these with scores on
the symptoms making up each of the syndromes.

Liddle's table of correlations is shown in Table 6.2. It can be seen that positive
symptoms (reality distortion) were not significantly correlated with performance
on any of the tests, but that both disorganisation and negative symptoms were
associated with impairment on some of them. Additionally, the patterns of
correlations were substantially different across the two syndromes: the negative
syndrome was correlated with poor performance on a test of long-term memory
(recognising names of famous people), a naming test and also two tests of
conceptual thinking (similarities and object classification). On the other hand,
disorganisation was correlated with impairment on orientation, sustained attention
(cancelling e's), one of two standard tests of short-term memory (Corsi block span)
and a different long-term memory test (word recognition memory).

Liddle did not actually include any executive tests in his test battery, but he
rectified this omission in a subsequent study (Liddle and Morris, 1991). This time
he rated symptoms and administered four executive tests, the Stroop test, the
Modified Wisconsin Card Sorting Test,[3] verbal fluency for letters and the Trail
Making Test, to a new group of forty-three chronic schizophrenic patients. The
findings are also shown in Table 6.2. Once again, both negative symptoms and
disorganisation, but not positive symptoms, showed significant correlations with
some of the test scores, and the pattern of correlations differed between the two
syndromes. Negative symptoms correlated with verbal fluency and Stroop

---

[3] A simplified form of the original test using less cards and in which the changes in sorting rule are announced.

Table 6.2 The neuropsychological correlates of positive, negative and disorganisation syndromes in schizophrenic patients

	Positive	Disorganisation	Negative
(a) Non-executive tests (from Liddle, 1987b, reproduced with permission)			
Orientation	−0.04	−0.31*	−0.29
Vocabulary	0.00	−0.18	−0.20
Cancelling e's	0.02	−0.48**	0.00
Digit span	0.04	0.01	−0.06
Corsi blocks	0.05	−0.38*	−0.02
Sentence repetition	0.04	0.23	−0.04
Word learning	−0.22	−0.36*	−0.02
Face learning	0.16	−0.13	−0.30
Long term memory	−0.08	−0.18	−0.51***
Object naming	−0.12	0.04	−0.40*
Similarities	0.06	−0.03	−0.36*
Object classification	0.00	−0.27	−0.38*
Figure ground perception	−0.18	−0.09	−0.30
(b) Executive tests (from Liddle and Morris, 1991, reproduced with permission)			
Verbal fluency	−0.01	−0.50**	−0.48**
Stroop Test	0.16	−0.36*	−0.40*
Trail Making Test (B)	−0.11	−0.58**	−0.13
Modified WCST	−0.17	−0.47**	−0.13

Note: * p < 0.05; ** p < 0.01; *** p < 0.001

performance, but not with performance on the modified Wisconsin Card Sorting Test or the Trail Making Test (at least part B, the part which requires executive function). Disorganisation was also correlated with verbal fluency and Stroop performance, but additionally with the Trail Making Test part B and the modified Wisconsin Card Sorting Test. Controlling for various potential confounding factors, both clinical (severity and chronicity of illness) and neuropsychological (slowness and general test performance as measured by performance on a naming test) made only minor differences to the pattern of correlations. Liddle and Morris concluded that the negative syndrome was particularly associated with impairment in those aspects of executive function governing the self-directed generation of mental activity, whereas disorganisation might reflect a specific difficulty in inhibiting inappropriate responses.

This was a bold conclusion, particularly when Liddle's (1987b) own earlier finding of significant correlations with non-executive tests had already raised the spectre of neuropsychological non-specificity. However, the claim is easy to examine further, as there have been over twenty more studies of the neuropsychological correlates of Liddle's three syndromes, and these have employed a wide variety of different tests. These studies are summarised in Table 6.3, from which it is apparent that, while many studies have found significant correlations between disorganisation and executive impairment, there have also been significant correlations with a number of other tests. Memory and general intellectual function are at least as well represented as executive function, and correlations have been found with impairment in sustained attention, language and visual perception. Within executive function itself, impairment on the Stroop test appears to be more frequently associated with disorganisation than with negative symptoms, and the reverse may be true for verbal fluency, but otherwise there is little to support Liddle and Morris' contention that the two syndromes show associations with different patterns of impairment.

Liddle's studies and those which followed seem to point an association between the disorganisation syndrome (and the negative syndrome) and some nonspecific cognitive factor, most obviously identifiable as general intellectual impairment. This does not exclude the possibility of an additional association with executive impairment (although it does beg the question of why the syndrome should be associated with both types of deficit). However, the problem is how to demonstrate this; as described in Chapter 4, general intellectual impairment will itself give rise to poor performance on specific neuropsychological tests, with the consequence that some or all of the correlations with executive impairment shown in Table 6.3 could be spurious.

Barrera *et al.* (2004) have recently carried out one of the very few studies that took steps to minimise the confounding effects of general intellectual impairment. They examined executive function in two groups of chronic schizophrenic patients, fifteen with thought disorder (defined as a global rating of moderate or greater on the TLC scale) and sixteen who showed no more than minimal degrees of the symptom (global TLC rating of absent or questionable). Seventeen normal controls were also tested. All the patients were selected on the basis that they were relatively intellectually intact, according to the criterion of having a current WAIS IQ of 85 or greater, i.e within one standard deviation of the normal population mean. The two patient groups and the normal controls were matched for age and NART-estimated premorbid IQ. The thought-disordered and non-thought-disordered patients were also well matched for current IQ.

All subjects were administered six executive tests. These included three 'second generation' executive tests, designed to overcome well-known problems with standard tests such as the Wisconsin Card Sorting Test, or to capture aspects of the dysexecutive syndrome not tapped by earlier tests. The Brixton test (Burgess and Shallice, 1997) was designed to cover the same conceptual ground as the

Table 6.3 Significant neuropsychological correlations with positive, negative and disorganisation syndromes in different studies of schizophrenic patients

	Positive	Disorganisation	Negative
Executive function			
WCST		✓[3] ✓[19] ✓[5] ✓[22] ✓[23] ✓[6] ✓[21] ✓[18] ✓[24] ✓[9]	✓[12] ✓[13] ✓[4] ✓[17] ✓[24] ✓[9]
Verbal fluency	✓[9]	✓[3] ✓[9] ✓[2] ✓[16]	✓[3] ✓[12] ✓[13] ✓[19] ✓[4] ✓[23] ✓[16] ✓[17] ✓[9]
Stroop test	✓[10]	✓[3] ✓[14] ✓[22] ✓[10] ✓[26]	✓[3] ✓[7]
Trailmaking test (B)		✓[3] ✓[18] ✓[22] ✓[23] ✓[9]	✓[13] ✓[19] ✓[4] ✓[23] ✓[9]
Short-term memory			
Digit span		✓[18] ✓[22] ✓[4] ✓[20]	✓[8] ✓[21]
Corsi blocks		✓[1]	
Long-term memory			
General memory		✓[15]	✓[13]
Verbal memory	✓[12]	✓[1] ✓[8] ✓[18] ✓[25]	✓[12] ✓[13] ✓[19] ✓[17]
Visual memory		✓[12] ✓[13]	✓[8] ✓[13] ✓[19] ✓[17]
Other		✓[2]	✓[1]
Working memory		✓[23] ✓[24]	✓[23]
General intellectual function			
Full scale IQ		✓[13] ✓[19]	✓[13]
Verbal IQ		✓[8]	✓[8]
Performance IQ			✓[17]
Other IQ		✓[7] ✓[8] ✓[2]	✓[1] ✓[2] ✓[7]
Miscellaneous			
Language		✓[8]	✓[1]
Visual/visuospatial function			✓[11]
Sustained attention		✓[1] ✓[18] ✓[2] ✓[21]	✓[19] ✓[18] ✓[2] ✓[21]

Notes:
WCST – Wisconsin Card Sorting Test.
[1] Liddle (1987b)
[2] Frith *et al.* (1991)
[3] Liddle and Morris (1991)
[4] Brown and White (1992)
[5] Van der Does *et al.* (1993)
[6] Bell *et al.* (1994)
[7] Brekke *et al.* (1995)
[8] Cuesta and Peralta (1995)
[9] Himelhoch *et al.* (1996)
[10] Joyce *et al.* (1996)
[11] Cadenhead *et al.* (1997)
[12] Norman *et al.* (1997)
[13] Basso *et al.* (1998)
[14] Baxter and Liddle (1998)
[15] Clark and O'Carroll (1998)
[16] Robert *et al.* (1998)
[17] Mohamed *et al.* (1999)
[18] Eckman and Shean (2000)/Rowe and Shean (1997)
[19] O'Leary *et al.* (2000)
[20] Tabares *et al.* (2000)
[21] Guillem *et al.* (2001)
[22] Moritz *et al.* (2001)
[23] Cameron *et al.* (2002)
[24] Daban *et al.* (2002)
[25] Pollice *et al.* (2002)
[26] Woodward *et al.* (2003)

Wisconsin Card Sorting Test; it requires the subject to predict where a blue spot will move to in an array of ten empty circles following a rule which changes unpredictably from time to time. In the The Hayling Sentence Completion Test (Burgess and Shallice, 1997) the subject has to complete sentences with a word that is unconnected to the sentence in every way; for example *The captain wanted to stay with the sinking –*, for which a correct reply might be 'light bulb'. It is similar to the Stroop test in that subjects have to inhibit a natural response. The Six Elements Test (Wilson *et al.*, 1996) is designed to provide an 'everyday' or 'ecologically valid' measure of executive impairment. It requires subjects to organise their activities in order to carry out parts of six tasks in a limited time period and without breaking certain rules. The other executive tests, verbal fluency for animals and words beginning with the letter S, and the Cognitive Estimates Test (Shallice and Evans, 1978), are described in Box 6.1.

The findings are shown in Figure 6.1. The thought-disordered patients performed significantly more poorly than the non-thought-disordered patients on all the executive tests apart from the verbal fluency tests. They were also impaired compared with the normal controls on all but one of the tasks (one of the two verbal fluency tasks). The non-thought-disordered patients also showed some degree of poorer performance than the normal controls on most of the tasks, but the differences only reached significance on one of these, the Six Elements Test.

Barrera *et al.'s* study does finally suggest that when measures are taken to reduce the noise introduced by general intellectual impairment – as well as possibly that produced by using an earlier generation of executive tests – thought disorder emerges as quite broadly and strongly associated with impaired executive function. The findings are not by any means decisive, as there was no relationship with verbal fluency, and the possibility of additional associations with non-executive test performance is not ruled out (although further results discussed in the next chapter go some way to dealing with this objection).

Conclusion

At the beginning of this chapter a distinction was drawn between on the one hand a set of changes in behaviour, the frontal lobe syndrome, and on the other hand a purely cognitive construct, the dysexecutive syndrome. This distinction may or may not ultimately be meaningful, and it has certainly been largely ignored in schizophrenia research, but it has the virtue that it provides a useful way of summarising the evidence.

The frontal lobe hypothesis of thought disorder has to overcome the obstacle that neurological accounts of the frontal lobe syndrome are not noteworthy for their descriptions of anything resembling thought disorder. However, close

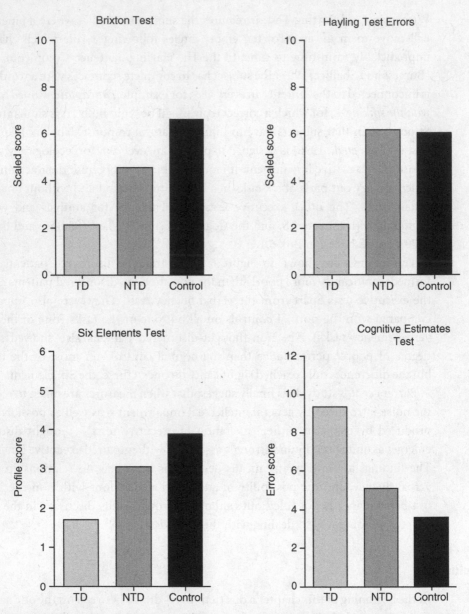

Figure 6.1   Performance of thought-disordered and non-thought-disordered schizophrenic patients and normal controls on four executive tests. Findings for the two fluency tests are not shown but did not distinguish the patient groups (from Barrera *et al*., 2004)

scrutiny of the literature does reveal evidence that the speech and language disorders such patients show go beyond a mere reduction and simplification of speech and reproduce some of the phenomena of thought disorder – if not faithfully, then closely enough to make schizophrenia researchers think they may be on the right track. Some frontal lobe patients digress from the topic, free associate, get distracted by irrelevant associations and produce narratives that do not hang together. They also appear to show something akin to word approximations and stiltedness. But even when it is at its most severe, this form of frontal speech perhaps does not capture the full richness and bizarreness of schizophrenic thought disorder.

In contrast to the essentially observational nature of studies on frontal lobe patients, investigation of the dysexecutive theory of thought disorder has been all hard-headed empirical investigation. The studies are a long way from being decisive and have not as yet succeeded in clearing all the methodological hurdles, but there is enough to suggest that there is an association – albeit not a particularly pure one – between thought disorder and dysexecutive syndrome.

7

The dyssemantic hypothesis of thought disorder

If the dysexecutive theory of thought disorder can be said to have a psychological rival, it is the idea that the symptom reflects some kind of disturbance in semantic memory. This approach has a longer history than the dysexecutive theory; in fact its origins go back to a time when the term semantic memory did not exist. Since the 'semantic' of semantic memory refers to meaning, it also has obvious points of continuity with the theme of semantic abnormality which emerged from the consideration of linguistic and pragmatic abnormalities in Chapters 4 and 5. The theoretical construct of semantic memory even comes with a simple operational process, malfunction of which seems almost tailor-made for giving rise to disorganisation of speech. This process is spreading activation, and the malfunction is the so-called semantic hyperpriming theory of thought disorder.

This chapter could be just about semantic hyperpriming. There is certainly a sizeable enough body of experimental evidence devoted to it. But increased semantic priming was not the first, nor the last, of what might be termed the dyssemantic hypotheses of thought disorder. As the 'dys' has meant quite different things in these theories, and since semantic memory is itself a somewhat fragmented concept – which has drawn on linguistics and computer science and even Aristotlean philosophy, as well as psychology and neuropsychology – the appropriate place to begin is with an account of what semantic memory is believed to be.

What is semantic memory?

Semantic memory refers quite simply to stored knowledge about the world. The concept first achieved wide currency when Tulving (1972) drew attention to a distinction that seemed to exist between two meanings of the term memory. One of these was episodic memory, or memory in the normally understood sense of the term: memory for personally experienced events, individual happenings and doings, such as what one had for breakfast and who one met on holiday last year. The other sense of the term referred to another large store of information, which like episodic memory is held outside consciousness but is capable of being retrieved into it. Tulving (1972) originally defined this as memory for the use of language, a kind of mental thesaurus of organised knowledge a person possesses about words and other verbal symbols, their meaning and referents and the relations among them.

Although Tulving (1983) accepted that the two memory stores were related, and probably interacted with each other all the time, he enumerated a number of basic differences in the characteristics of the knowledge they held. For example, episodic memories are always remembered as involving the rememberer, and they always appear in conscious awareness accompanied by some specification of the time and place at which they occurred, even if this is only vague. In contrast, the basic units of semantic memory are impersonal – items of shared factual knowledge which are held without any connotations of 'it happened to me' or 'I did that.' Also, unlike episodic memory, which is organised linearly along a continuum of personal time, all information in semantic memory exists embedded within a network of inter-connected knowledge.

Since Tulving's original definition, the concept of semantic memory has been extended without demur to encompass all knowledge (Kintsch, 1980; Tulving, 1983). This ranges from knowledge of the meaning of words, to general know-ledge, such as knowing the capital of France and the chemical formula for salt, to such abstract concepts as truth and justice. Also held in semantic memory are the complicated sets of social rules referred to as schemas, frames or scripts, which are necessary for doing things like ordering a meal in a restaurant.

A further subcomponent of semantic memory is personal semantic memory – knowledge about oneself, rather than the world. The most basic item of personal semantic information is knowing one's name, but this class of knowledge extends to all kinds of personal data, such as where one lived at different times of one's life, what books one has read, and even to what food one likes to order in the aforementioned restaurants.

Despite its obvious importance, understanding of semantic memory remains, as Baddeley (1990) noted, somewhat fragmentary and lacking in coherence. It is widely assumed that the store is organised in the form of a network, so that particular items of knowledge, or nodes as they are often called, are linked to one another depending on the existence of an association between them. For example the concept of *bird* is associated with concepts relating to its defining features, such as having feathers, being able to fly, etc. There is also a hierarchical element to this organisation, so that *bird* is linked upwards to the superordinate category of *animals*, and also downwards to specific examples of birds, both typical, such as *robin* and *canary*, and atypical, such as *ostrich*. This configuration of horizontal and vertical associations constitutes the meaning of *bird*.

As Baddeley (1990) also noted, the network theory of semantic memory is ultimately traceable all the way back to Aristotle's efforts to define words logically, but it owes a larger theoretical debt to computer science. In particular, all such models derive ultimately from an attempt by Quillian (1966; 1969) to develop a method of storing semantic information in a computer, in such a way as to enable the verification of simple propositions like *a canary can fly* and *a canary has skin*. In order to minimise the amount of space needed for storage, Quillian proposed that the features relevant to a particular concept were stored at the highest level of the hierarchy to which they were generally applicable. Thus, information which is true of birds in general, such as they can fly and have feathers, need not be stored as a link to the nodes for every different kind of bird. Instead, the fact that a canary can fly can be verified by establishing that there is a link between *canary* and *bird*, and between *bird* and *can fly*. Since an ostrich cannot fly, this information is stored as a link to the node for *ostrich*.

If such an organising principle also characterised human semantic memory then verifying the proposition that *Canaries can fly* should take longer than *A canary is a bird* or *A canary is yellow*. This is because the verification involves two stages, first establishing that canaries are birds and second that birds can fly, and so the links between two nodes have to be traversed rather than just one.

This prediction was supported in a famous study by Collins and Quillian (1969). They found that normal subjects took progressively longer to verify sentences such as *A maple is a maple*, *An oak has acorns* and *A birch has seeds*, as the verification required moving between no, one or two hierarchical levels. However, they also found that this relationship did not hold true for false sentences; it took no longer to decide that *Coca-cola is blue* is untrue, where a direct link exists to the property of colour, than *Lemonade is alcoholic*, where the contradiction concerns the properties of soft drinks in general.

Other studies produced further inconsistent findings. Important among these was the fact that the original model implied all links were equal in strength,[1] but it could be demonstrated that typical examples of a category were verified more quickly than atypical ones. Thus subjects responded 'true' faster to the statement *A canary is a bird* than to *An ostrich is a bird*. This led Collins and Loftus (1975) to produce a revised model which introduced, among other things, the concepts of semantic distance and spreading activation. Closely related concepts were now considered to be closer to each other in the semantic network and more distantly related ones further away. Verification of statements was no longer just a matter of establishing whether or not a link existed between two nodes, but also depended on an outward spread of activation from each of them, which then either intersected or

---

[1] According to Collins and Loftus (1975) this is not strictly true and is a misunderstanding based on the simplified version of the model presented in the Collins and Quillian (1969) study.

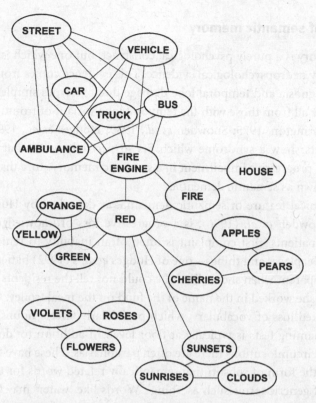

Figure 7.1   Schematic representation of concept relatedness in a semantic network. A shorter line represents greater relatedness (From Collins and Loftus, 1975, copyright © 1975 by the American Psychological Association. Reprinted with permission).

failed to intersect. Collins and Loftus' diagram of a hypothetical fragment of semantic memory is reproduced in Figure 7.1.

This network model of semantic memory can be and has been given layers of secondary complication, but the hypothesis of spreading activation remains firmly entrenched in psychological thinking. When a node is activated, by hearing or reading it or thinking about it and also – of particular relevance in the present context – when preparing to speak about it, other nodes become activated as well, with the degree of activation being proportional to the semantic distance between them. Thus, for example, the word *robin* will activate the nodes for *bird*; plus other typical examples of birds, such as *sparrow*; and also its features, such as *feathers* and *red breast*. These associated units remain activated for a finite period of time, of the order of milliseconds. Nodes for less closely related concepts, for example *ostrich* and *has skin* may be too distant to be activated, but there may still be spread of activation to them if they have already been activated by, say, a question containing both words.

The neuropsychology of semantic memory

Semantic memory is a purely psychological construct, but one which is strikingly corroborated by neuropsychological evidence. This evidence comes from patients with aphasia, agnosia and temporal lobe damage due to herpes simplex encephalitis, but above all from those with the temporal lobe variant of fronto-temporal dementia (Warrington, 1975; Snowden *et al.*, 1989; Hodges *et al.*, 1992). Many of these patients show a syndrome which fits so perfectly with what would be predicted from progressive impairment in a semantic memory store that it is now universally known as semantic dementia.

The core clinical feature of semantic dementia, as described by Hodges *et al.* (1992) and Snowden *et al.* (1996), is a progressive loss of knowledge of word meaning. The patients' first complaint is often of an inability to remember the names of people, places and things – one of Hodges *et al.*'s (1992) patient's illness first became apparent when she realised she could not tell the residents of the old people's home she worked in the name of the food on the meal trolley. On testing there is a marked loss of vocabulary, which particularly affects nouns, and performance on naming tests is typically at floor level. In addition to 'don't know' responses and circumlocutions there are often paraphasias. These have the feature that they take the form of substituting semantically related words for the correct one and use of generic terms such as 'thing'. Words like 'water' may be used to refer to all forms of liquid, including tea and orange juice.

The problem is not just one of naming. A lack of knowledge about the words can be demonstrated by asking patients to sort pictures of animals and manmade objects into categories according to their attributes, e.g. whether they are large or small, domestic or foreign, electrical or non-electrical, etc. Many patients make multiple errors on this normally very simple task. They also perform poorly when asked to give definitions of words, with their responses often being grossly impoverished and containing elementary factual errors.

Whether the higher-order semantic structures of frames, schemas and scripts are affected has not been clearly established. However, Snowden *et al.* (1996) pointed to certain clinical features which could plausibly be understood in this way. Thus, patients tend to adopt a fixed routine, carrying out particular activities at particular times and becoming annoyed at any interruption or deviation from the schedule. One of Snowden *et al.*'s patients took to asking visitors what time they were going to leave as soon as they arrived and would remind them to do so at the allotted hour. Another, who became very preoccupied with odours, took to sniffing visitors if they were wearing perfume or aftershave, and approaching strangers in the street in order to smell them.

Although patients with semantic dementia often state that they cannot remember anything, memory in the conventional episodic sense remains well preserved. They continue to find their way around, keep appointments, and have no difficulty remembering day-to-day events.[2] Patients remain independent and carry on activities ranging from shopping and cooking to driving until late into the course of the disease. Other areas of cognitive function, such as arithmetical skills and visual and visuospatal abilities, are also remarkably preserved – one of Snowden *et al.*'s patients continued to be highly proficient in drawing and copying despite having severe difficulties in recognising the objects in them. Executive function is also said to be spared, although this can be difficult to test (Hodges and Patterson, 1997; Snowden, 1996).

As the disease progresses, speech becomes increasingly empty of information, and there is more use of stereotyped phrases like 'You don't realize, do you?', 'Well, it's one of those things' and 'I'll just have to check on it.' There is a gradual contraction in the topics of conversation, which focus exclusively on a few autobiographically relevant topics. Echolalia and perseveration start to appear or become more prominent. Ultimately only a few verbal stereotypies remain and then these too are lost, leading to mutism.

The first dyssemantic hypothesis: overinclusive thinking

After giving his pioneering account of the clinical features of thought disorder, as described in Chapter 1, Cameron (1939a,b) went on to try and capture the underlying psychological nature of some of them. To do this, he took five of the most severely thought-disordered patients from his original study, plus a comparison group of six patients with dementia, and gave them a task where they had to group twenty-two wooden blocks, varying in colour, shape, size and height, into four groups. The problem was not simple – there were five colours and six shapes, two different sizes and two different heights – but the experimenter continuously provided feedback in order to enable the subject to acquire the correct solution, which was large high, large flat, small high and small flat blocks.

Both the schizophrenic and the demented patients appeared to have difficulty grasping the abstract nature of the sorting principle and ignoring the individual features of the blocks, such as their colour. However, whereas the demented patients were rigid and repetitive, the schizophrenic patients were versatile and flexible. They also showed a tendency to incorporate all kinds of irrelevant material into their solutions. Observing the investigator taking notes, one patient said, 'That pencil is yellow so it ought to be in the game.' When another patient was

---

[2] However, this preservation may not be complete. Graham and Hodges (1997) have found that, while the patients remember recent events well, their memory for remote personal events typically shows marked impairment.

questioned about a grouping he had made, he answered, 'These are kept in a box together', and pointed to the test material box across the table. A particularly graphic example of this phenomenon, which also revealed how closely it was bound up with thought disorder, occurred when a patient's attention was directed to the fact that he had put a green triangle in with three blue blocks of various shapes. He looked at the group, and said slowly and earnestly:

Three blues! Now how about the green blotter? Put it in there too. Peas you eat – you can't eat them unless you write on it [indicating the blotter]. You've got to turn that blotter into peas before you can prove you can't eat them. Like that wrist-watch [on Cameron's wrist, beyond the blotter] – I don't see any three meals coming off that watch.

Cameron (1939b) used the term 'overinclusiveness' to refer to this failure to confine thinking to a single frame of reference, and proposed it as a unifying explanation for his descriptive abnormalities of asyndetic thinking, metonymic distortion and interpenetration of themes.

Had the term semantic memory been in existence in 1939, Cameron would almost certainly have identified it as the site of the hypothesised breakdown in conceptual thinking which gave rise to asyndetic thinking. It probably also would not have escaped him that semantic memory was the repository not only for concepts but also for knowledge of the meanings of words, and so offered a natural way of extending the theory to account for his metonymic distortion or word approximations. Had he somehow had access to the very recent literature on personal semantic memory, he might even have been able to incorporate interpenetration of themes into his theory of overinclusiveness, as a breakdown of the boundary between personal and impersonal conceptual knowledge.

As it was, Cameron did not take his theory of overinclusive thinking very far and never made any attempt to test it. Others, however, were not deterred. When Payne (1960) reviewed the field, he was able to report on fifteen studies, all of which found evidence of overinclusiveness in schizophrenia, sometimes using quite ingenious ways of measuring this. For example, Zaslow (1950) showed schizophrenic patients and controls a series of cards, the first of which showed a triangle and the last a circle, with the shape changing progressively from one to the other in the intervening cards. When asked to indicate where the triangles and the circles ended, the schizophrenic patients included more cards in both categories. Chapman and Taylor (1957) required schizophrenic patients and controls to sort cards with words like apple and fish on them into categories such as fruit. The normal subjects made virtually no errors, but, while the schizophrenic patients excluded completely unrelated words, they included significant numbers of incorrect but related words, such as vegetables. Finally, in what became a standard test, Moran (1953) and Epstein (1953) presented schizophrenic patients and controls with a stimulus word; the subjects then had to underline which of a list of other words were integral to the concept of it (e.g. House: *walls*, curtains, telephone, bricks, *roof*). The schizophrenic patients included significantly more of the distantly related words as essential parts of the concept of the stimulus word.

By the time Payne reviewed the field again in 1973, the trickle of studies had become a flood. A large number of studies of overinclusive thinking, using an only slightly smaller number of different tasks, had been carried out, and on balance overinclusiveness still had the benefit of more positive than negative replications. Payne pooled the data from studies using three tests, including the above Moran/ Epstein test, which his own work had suggested were the best measures of over-inclusiveness. The 'combined overinclusion scores' derived from these three tests for a number of different patient groups are shown in Table 7.1. Acute schizo-phrenic patients showed levels of overinclusiveness that were on average twice as high as those for normal subjects. The scores of manic patients were, if anything, even higher. However this did not hold true for chronic schizophrenic patients, whose scores were only marginally higher than those of normal subjects. A small group of patients with organic brain disease also showed overinclusiveness, and it was also clear that some patients with alcoholism, neurosis and personality dis-order were more overinclusive than normal subjects.

As Table 7.1 indicates, Payne (1973) found no difference between the over-inclusiveness scores of paranoid and nonparanoid schizophrenic patients, a com-parison which at the time was de rigeur in psychological studies of schizophrenia. He interpreted this to mean that overinclusive thinking was not associated with delusions, since these were the characteristic symptom of paranoid schizophrenia. Payne and everyone else at the time also assumed that overinclusiveness was associated with thought disorder; this assumption, however, was only ever put to the test in a single study. Hawks and Payne (1971) administered their three tests of overinclusiveness to thirty-six acute admissions with a clinical diagnosis of schizophrenia, plus eighteen patients with other diagnoses (mainly with neurotic and personality diagnoses, but including two with mania) and eighteen normal controls. All the groups were matched for age and IQ. Beforehand, eighteen of the schizophrenic patients had been independently categorised as showing thought disorder,[3] and eighteen as not showing the symptom. The thought-disordered schizophrenic patients were found to have a significantly higher mean combined overinclusion score than the non-thought-disordered schizophrenic patients, who

---

[3] Strictly, they were considered to show 'overinclusive thought disorder', defined as: 'The patient describes interference or distraction while trying to think along objective lines...loses thread of thoughts...unwarranted or irrelevant thoughts drift into mind...concentration sometimes impaired by interfering thoughts...distracted by outside stimuli, while trying to concentrate...unable to attend at times because distracted by silly details.'

Table 7.1 Combined overinclusion scores in different patient groups

(From Payne, 1973)

Group	Mean	S.D.
Paranoid schizophrenics (N = 38)	8.70	3.74
Non-paranoid schizophrenics (N = 55)	8.98	4.07
Acute undifferentiated schizophrenics (N = 20)	10.05	4.50
Chronic schizophrenics (N = 17)	5.33	2.43
Manics (N = 13)	10.92	4.62
Depressives (N = 41)	6.32	2.98
Organics (N = 7)	11.57	3.46
Alcoholics (N = 12)	8.00	2.86
Character disorders (N = 20)	7.10	2.95
Extraverted neurotics (N = 12)	8.58	3.46
Introverted neurotics (N = 20)	6.95	2.71
Combined neurotic group (N = 55)	7.29	2.93
Normals (N = 20)	4.90	1.58

did not differ from the non-schizophrenic patients or the normal controls. The correlations between overinclusiveness and other symptoms in the whole group of fifty-four patients are shown in Table 7.2. There were few significant correlations with delusions; only that with ideas of influence reached significance. On the other hand, overinclusiveness correlated significantly with scores for thought disorder, as well as with a number of other symptoms, including talkativeness, verbal responsiveness, increased motor activity and hostility, which might with greater or lesser degrees of plausibility be regarded as associated with this.

Table 7.2 Correlations between combined overinclusion scores and symptoms in fifty-four patients

(From Hawks and Payne, 1971)

Symptom	Correlation
Ideas of influence	0.26*
Ideas of reference	0.09
Ideas of persecution	0.27
Ideas of grandeur	0.04
Hypochondriacal delusions	−0.19
Open hostility	0.36*
Motor activity	0.29*
Talkativeness	0.45**
Motor speed	0.32*
Verbal responsiveness	0.36**
Thought disorder[1]	−0.30*

Notes: *P < 0.05; **P < 0.01.
[1] Although the correlation appears to be in the wrong direction, in the text it is stated that overinclusiveness and thought disorder were significantly positively correlated. Possibly this was an artefact of the way the symptom was rated.

For Payne, overinclusive thinking seemed to have all the right qualifications for a psychological abnormality underlying and perhaps giving rise to thought disorder. He concluded that it was a somewhat elusive and relatively uncommon phenomenon which appeared to be present in about a third of patients with acute schizophrenia, and could also be seen in mania, but was not characteristic of chronic schizophrenia. It tended to occur in patients who were talkative, overactive, verbally responsive and hostile and who were judged clinically to be thought disordered. Yet, even as Payne made this statement, research into overinclusive thinking was coming to a halt. According to Chapman and Chapman (1973) this was mainly due to criticisms of the three measures Payne relied on to calculate his combined overinclusion score, some of which were justified but others of which appear to have been mere psychometric nitpicking. The occasional study of overinclusive thinking has been carried out since then (Andreasen and Powers, 1974; see also Harrow and Quinlan, 1985), and the term can occasionally be spotted in psychiatric textbooks, where it is often used wrongly as a descriptive term for thought disorder. But research has moved on, indifferent to the fact that, as Chapman and Chapman noted, overinclusive thinking is the only psychological abnormality ever found to be more characteristic of acute schizophrenia than chronic schizophrenia.

Thought disorder as increased semantic priming

Approximately ten years after the demise of overinclusiveness, Maher (1983) advanced what he called 'a tentative theory of schizophrenic utterance'. Notable for its simplicity and originality, this also held out the rather dizzying prospect that an arcane theoretical process originally derived from computer science might provide a key to understanding one of the symptoms of a major, putatively brain-based mental illness. His proposal was essentially that thought disorder was due to increased spreading activation in semantic memory.[4] Although dyssemantic in all but name, the theory was all the more remarkable for the fact that Maher managed to avoid using the terms semantic memory or spreading activation throughout the course of what was a quite lengthy theoretical account.

Simplified, re-arranged slightly and rephrased in the terminology of semantic memory, Maher's argument ran as follows. Hearing or speaking a word, or intending to speak it, activates associations that have been acquired to that word, giving them the potential for entering consciousness for a limited period of time. Or in other words, when a cognitive process activates a node in semantic memory, this increases the probability that some of the nodes with links to it will be activated as well. Normally, most of these associations do not enter consciousness. Were they to do so, the conduct of normal speech would become extremely difficult. For example, in the sentence *Bees make honey*, associations to the word bee might include sting, wasp and hive, and those to honey might include sweet and comb. Were such associations to be routinely incorporated into speech, the sentences which resulted, such as *Bees make sweet*, would strike the listener as distinctly odd. Therefore, in Maher's words, 'we might conceive of the utterance of a complete and organised sentence as a feat achieved by the effective exclusion of the associations that lie like a web of distractions around each element in the sentence'.

Even so, Maher argued, such activated associations did sometimes intrude into normal speech when they happened to serve the speaker's purpose. He himself had collected a number of examples of this phenomenon, including: 'A career in art has *drawbacks*'; 'This book, written by a man awaiting execution in Sing Sing prison, is quite *electrifying*'; 'China: a giant *peeking* cautiously at the world'; and ' "Lamp at midnight," to put it plainly, had a touch of greatness, catching a moment of irreconcilable conflict in Catholic Church history with a *burning* eloquence worthy of the vast and timeless issues *at stake*.'[5]

---

[4] The theory was in fact more complicated than this, proposing a further abnormal process involving defective attentional control of speech.

[5] Ironically these last two examples were drawn from the notebooks of the arch-behaviourist, Skinner.

Experimental evidence for spread of activation from words to their associations was available from the so-called lexical decision task. In this, subjects see a string of letters flashed up on a screen and have to decide by a key press whether it is a word or a non-word. Immediately beforehand, a word – the prime – is briefly shown, which may or may not be semantically related to the target word (if this happens to be a real word). The time taken to decide whether the target is a real word is significantly reduced when the prime is related to the target. This facilitation, or the semantic priming effect as it went on to become known as, can be explained as the prime producing spread of activation to the target, and hence reducing the degree of activation subsequently needed to allow the verification that it is a real word to take place.

The period of time over which the prime facilitates lexical decision is short, typically of the order of less than a second. In addition, it is highly probable that more than one process underlies the effect. Thus Maher pointed out that activation could either spread to all the words associated with a particular word, or be constrained to only those words appropriate to the context. For example, in the sentence, *He sold his stock because his broker advised him to do so*, does activation spread only to share, bond, dividend, etc., or does it also spread to associations having to do with livestock, inventory, theatre, and so on? Maher cited evidence from priming studies suggesting that both processes occur; initially there is activation to all associations, but that to context-irrelevant meanings decays quite rapidly, whereas that to context-relevant associations lasts longer.

Maher was now in a position to articulate his theory. If the associative process – i.e. spreading activation – in schizophrenia was larger in magnitude and/or persisted longer than normal, this could cause an intrusion of material into speech that would normally be excluded on the basis of its irrelevance to the topic. Depending on the severity of the disturbance it is easy to see how the result might be speech that was merely richer than usual in associations of the type described above, or, at the other extreme, speech that was strewn with multiple intrusions which seriously compromised its intelligibility.

The semantic network itself was normal in this theory; the problem was not one of abnormal associations, but the inappropriate intrusion of normal associations into speech. However, Maher considered it quite possible that the repeated experience of intrusions might lead to the links between concepts being remodelled, and so it would not be surprising if over time patients developed idiosyncratic and bizarre associations.

Unlike Cameron, Maher lost no time in putting his theory to experimental test, and for this it was natural to turn to the lexical decision task. He and his co-workers (Manschreck *et al.*, 1988) examined twelve chronic schizophrenic patients with thought disorder, twelve without this symptom, and eleven normal controls. Presence of thought disorder was based on a score of 3 or greater out of 5 on one or more of the items of understandability, derailment, logic, poverty of information conveyed and neologisms. The groups were matched for age and the patient groups had similar lengths of illness. However, the schizophrenic patients had significantly less years of education than the controls.

The patients and controls were given fifty trials, in which the target was an associated word, a non-associated word, or a nonword. Setting a trend for future studies, Manschreck *et al.* introduced their own variation on the standard procedure; in this case some of the primes were nonwords as well. The interval between onset of the prime and onset of the target (commonly referred to as the stimulus onset asynchrony or SOA), was short at 250ms.

Measures of accuracy of identification of words did not distinguish the three groups. As shown in Figure 7.2a, all three groups also showed significant priming, i.e. their mean reaction time to primed words was significantly shorter than that to unprimed words. However, whereas the degree of priming was similar in the normal controls and the non-thought-disordered schizophrenic patients (37ms vs. 36ms), at 83ms it was more than twice as great in the thought-disordered patients.

Manschreck's study was marred by the fact that the thought-disordered patients were on average faster to respond than the controls in both the primed and unprimed conditions, a result that runs counter to the almost universal finding that patients with schizophrenia as a group are slow on reaction time tasks. Further studies followed, one of the best-known of which was carried out by Spitzer *et al.* (1993) on fifty schizophrenic patients and fifty controls. They used a procedure similar to that of Manschreck *et al.* (1988) but tested subjects at both a short SOA (200ms) and a long SOA (700ms). This was in recognition of the increasing evidence that at least two processes were involved in the priming effect, as hinted at by Maher (1983). One of these was the rapid, automatic process of spreading activation seen at short SOAs, and the other was a slower, more controlled, but not necessarily more conscious process where the subject uses the nature of the prime to generate an 'expectancy set' of potential targets. When the patient group was split according to scores on the thought disorder item of the Brief Psychiatric Rating Scale, it was apparent, as shown in Figure 7.2b, that there was significantly greater priming in the thought-disordered patients than the non-thought-disordered patients. The difference between the thought-disordered and non-thought-disordered patients was significant at the long SOA, but was only at trend level for the short SOA.

In this study, in contrast to that of Manschreck *et al.* the schizophrenic patients were overall significantly slower than the controls on all components of the lexical decision task. Although reassuring, this result brings its own complications. If schizophrenic patients are slower to respond on both the unprimed and primed versions of the task, the value for priming will be inflated merely for arithmetical

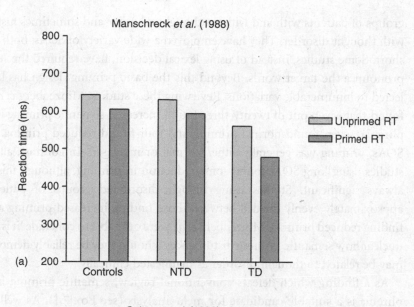

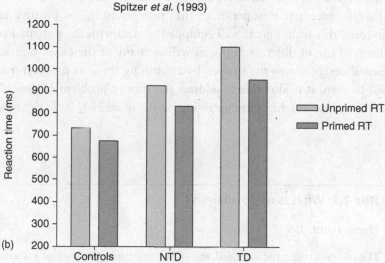

Figure 7.2   Semantic priming in two studies of schizophrenic patients (data from Spitzer *et al.*,1993 are for 200ms SOA, the findings were similar with 700ms SOA)

reasons – the difference between 900 and 600 is greater than that between 600 and 400, even though the proportional reduction is the same. Spitzer *et al.* controlled for this confounding factor by recalculating priming as the percentage gain in reaction time. This left the general pattern of the findings unchanged; however, the differences were now no longer significant at either SOA.

Many more studies of semantic priming in schizophrenia have been carried out. These have been carried out on unselected groups of schizophrenic patients, separate groups of patients with and without thought disorder and sometimes just patients with thought disorder. They have employed a wide variety of SOAs, both long and short. Some studies, instead of using lexical decision, have required the subjects to pronounce the target words. Beyond this the basic priming design has been subjected to innumerable variations. Reviewing these studies, Minzenberg *et al.* (2002) found that seven out of twenty-three found increased semantic priming in schizophrenia, seven found normal priming and four found reduced priming. At short SOAs, priming was generally either normal or increased. In contrast, all of seven studies using long SOAs found some reduction in priming, although this was not always significant. Studies using thought-disordered groups of patients were approximately evenly divided between those finding increased priming and those finding reduced priming. Minzenberg *et al.* were only able to conclude 'it is presently unclear how semantic priming disturbances (should they be reliably demonstrated) may be related to thought disorder as manifested clinically'.

As a finding which defeats conventional review, semantic priming in schizophrenia is a suitable candidate for meta-analysis (see Box 7.1). As well as being generally accepted as superior to the 'vote counting' of positive and negative findings, this technique is well equipped to deal with the potential confounding effects of use of different SOAs, as well as many of the other vagaries in experimental design across the studies, by examining them as moderator variables. As will be seen, it is also able to address the thorny problem of general slowing in reaction time in schizophrenia giving rise to spuriously large values for semantic priming.

Box 7.1 What is meta-analysis?

(From Hunt, 1997)

The review article, the standard way of summarising the state of a scientific area, is known to be a deeply flawed tool. As well as having no set rules, it is open to bias – reviews of the same set of studies can and regularly do reach diametrically opposed conclusions. Meta-analysis is simply a way of mathematically combining the results of studies in a particular area. It was invented in 1904 by the statistician Pearson, and modern techniques were later developed independently by Glass and Rosenthal.

Meta-analysis proceeds by extracting a summable measure of the difference under consideration in each study. The most widely used unit of measurement is the effect size (Cohen's *d*), the mean difference between the experimental and control group on the variable under study divided by the standard deviation of the whole sample. The effect sizes from all the studies are then averaged, using a formula which gives more weight to studies with larger sample sizes. In the biological sciences the rule of thumb for interpreting these pooled effect sizes is: 0.1–0.3 = small, 0.4–0.7 = medium and 0.8 or greater = large. If so wished, studies with extreme results, which might be distorting the overall effect size, can be identified and excluded to give a pooled effect size for a homogeneous set of studies.

Common sense, as well as a number of sound mathematical reasons, dictates that a meta-analysis should include as many studies as possible. Thus all potential studies need to be located and scrutinised, and often their authors contacted, to obtain the data necessary to permit effect sizes to be extracted. When this fails, as it usually does, publication bias – the tendency of small studies with negative findings not to get published and so influence the results – can be examined by means of a funnel plot. This is a graph of the individual effect sizes plotted against the sample size. Large studies produce effect sizes which are closer to the overall mean effect size than small ones, producing an inverted funnel shape. Absence of one of the tails – in other words a lack of studies with results contradictory to the main finding – indicates publication bias.

Contrary to the ever-popular 'apples and oranges' argument, findings from very different types of studies can and should be included in a meta-analysis. In fact this is one of the great advantages of the technique, since it allows questions about what influences or moderates the effect size to be asked in a mathematically rigorous way. It is thus a simple matter to test statistically whether the effect size is greater in men than in women, increases or decreases with the age of the subjects in the studies, is systematically affected by the different techniques employed in the studies and so on. Other commonly employed moderator variables include year of publication and overall quality of the study, but the range of these is limited only by human ingenuity.

Pomarol-Clotet *et al.* (unpublished) meta-analysed 24 published studies, plus a single unpublished study (Leeson *et al.*, unpublished). To be included studies had to report reaction time data on schizophrenic patients and normal controls in any type of semantic priming paradigm. These were used to calculate an overall effect size for the difference in the magnitude of semantic priming between schizophrenic patients as a group and normal controls. For the purpose of this analysis, when studies divided their schizophrenic samples into those with and without thought disorder, these were combined. Similarly, when studies examined priming at two or more SOAs, the effect sizes were averaged (these were then separated again for the analysis of moderator variables, below). Also ignored were the many variations in technique across the studies. A perhaps more fundamental methodological difference is whether the studies used a lexical decision task or a word pronunciation task. However, most of the studies used the former measure, and so the overall effect size was calculated first including the small number of word pronounciation studies and then calculated excluding these.

The pooled effect size from the 25 studies was +0.07 (CI −0.04/+0.18). The positive sign means that priming was in the direction of being increased in schizophrenia, but the fact that the confidence interval crosses zero means that it was not statistically significant. The data were significantly heterogeneous, but homogeneity was achieved by excluding four studies with outlying effect sizes; this made little difference to the pooled effect size, which became 0.01 (CI −0.11/+0.13). Excluding the two studies using pronunciation rather than lexical decision also made little difference. A funnel plot of the studies is shown in Figure 7.3; it is reasonably symmetrical suggesting that there is no publication bias.

However, the pooled effect size for the fifteen studies which compared thought-disordered schizophrenic patients with normal controls was +0.24 (CI +0.07/+0.40), indicating significantly increased priming. These studies were again heterogeneous, and the effect size climbed further to +0.55 (CI +0.36/+0.73) when five studies with outlying effect sizes were excluded. In contrast, pooling the twelve studies that compared non-thought-disordered patients with controls yielded an effect size of

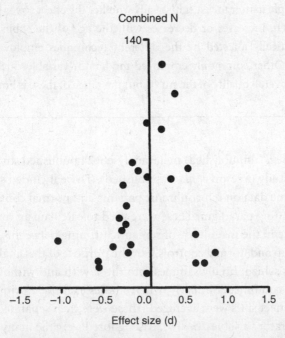

Figure 7.3   Funnel plot of 25 effect sizes for semantic priming in schizophrenia

+0.13 (CI +0.04/+0.29) for semantic priming, a non-significant finding. These studies were homogeneous.

Next SOA was examined as a moderator variable. For this studies were coded as employing a short SOA (≤400ms) or long SOA (>400ms). This yielded an effect size for 15 studies with short SOAs of +0.15 compared with –0.05 in 14 studies using long SOAs, a significant difference. (The larger number of studies in this analysis reflects the fact that some studies tested their subjects at both short and long SOAs.) In other words, any increased semantic priming in schizophrenia is due to an effect at short prime-target intervals only, and so reflects increased spreading activation rather than an increase in the slower controlled process or processes. This can be seen particularly clearly when the effect sizes for priming are plotted against the range of SOAs used in the studies (see Figure 7.4). When the SOA is very short (0–200 ms), no increase in priming is observed. As the SOA increases up to around 400 ms, the majority of studies have positive effect sizes, indicating increased semantic priming in schizophrenia. Beyond 800 ms, fewer studies have positive findings, and studies with large negative effect sizes start to appear.

Among the other moderator variables examined, age was not significant but duration of illness was – priming was greater with a shorter length of illness. There were too few studies carried out on groups of unmedicated patients to examine the effects of treatment.

The above analysis examined the difference in the degree of priming *between* schizophrenic patients and controls. As almost all the studies provided data on

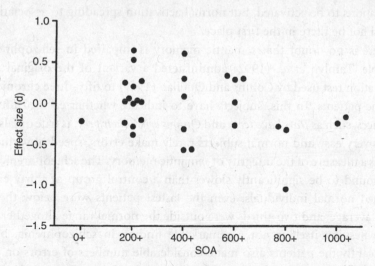

Figure 7.4   Effect sizes for semantic priming in schizophrenia in different studies plotted as a function of the stimulus onset asynchrony (SOA) used.

mean unprimed and primed reaction times in the two groups, it is also possible to calculate an effect size for the priming effect *within* each group. Like Spitzer *et al.*'s (1993) method of calculating priming in terms of percentage gain, this measure should be immune to the effects of general slowing of reaction time in schizophrenia. Pooling data for controls across 23 studies yielded an effect size for priming in normal subjects of 0.40. The corresponding effect size for priming in schizophrenic patients was not significantly different at 0.25. Significant differences did not appear when the comparison was restricted to studies using short SOAs, or to patients with thought disorder.

If one accepts the gospel according to meta-analysis, increased semantic priming is a genuine phenomenon in schizophrenia. The effect is restricted to patients with thought disorder and is most marked, or perhaps only evident, at short SOAs, and so reflects increased spreading activation rather than abnormality in a longer latency, controlled process or processes. However, meta-analysis is a two-edged sword: it singularly fails to exclude the possibility that some or all of the differences found might be due to the general slowing of reaction time in schizophrenia.

Thought disorder as disorganisation in the structure of semantic memory

For Maher (1983) the associative network was not intrinsically abnormal in thought-disordered schizophrenia, although he considered the possibility that it might become abnormal over time. But if the architecture of semantic memory were itself disorganised this might well have much the same disruptive effect on speech – it would be a case not of abnormal activation causing too-distant associations to be activated, but normal activation spreading to associations that should not be there in the first place.

There is no doubt that semantic memory is impaired in schizophrenia. For example, Tamlyn *et al.* (1992) administered a variant of the original sentence verification test used by Collins and Quillian (1969) to fifty-three chronic schizophrenic patients. In this, subjects have to indicate whether each of fifty simple sentences, such as *Rats have teeth* and *Onions crush their prey*, is true or false. As the task is very easy and normal subjects rarely make errors, speed of verification is used as a measure of the integrity of semantic memory. The schizophrenic patients were found to be significantly slower than a control group of thirty-eight age-matched normal individuals; even the fastest patients were below the control group average, and two-thirds were outside the normal range altogether.

Slowness by itself is not a remarkable finding in schizophrenia, but more significantly the patients also made considerable numbers of errors on the task: none of the controls made more than two errors, whereas fourteen (26%) of the patients made three or more verification errors, and five of them made more than ten errors. As shown in Table 7.3, these were often but not always in the direction of verifying false statements as true. While some patients gave no or facile reasons for their answers, the explanations of others showed illogicality, and in one or two cases clear instances of thought disorder were elicited.

It is less easy to show that the semantic memory deficit in schizophrenia is more than just part of the pattern of general poor neuropsychological performance that characterises the disorder. In Tamlyn *et al.*'s study poor performance on the 'silly sentences' was closely associated with general intellectual impairment. On the other hand, a few studies have documented poor semantic memory test performance in schizophrenic patients selected for meeting some criterion of overall intellectual intactness, either relatively loose (Clare *et al.*, 1993) or quite strict (McKay *et al.*, 1996). But whatever the truth of the matter is, it is not uncommon to encounter,

Table 7.3 Schizophrenic patients' explanations for their semantic errors

(From Tamlyn *et al.*, 1992)

Rats have teeth (replied false)
'Because I don't think they do have teeth.'
Pork chops come in long strands (replied true)
'Because it's true, because you can buy them at the butcher's.'
Owls have blades (replied true)
'To fly with.'
Captains are used for eating soup (replied true)
'To feed with – soup. I think they eat soup don't they, they don't get
    hungry – use him with a spoon.'
Screwdrivers have a profession (replied true)
'They do have a profession, people use them at work. People have a
    profession who use them, so they're used.'
Beefsteaks crawl on their bellies (replied true)
'A cow is still alive before it's slaughtered, so it could be true they
    could crawl on their bellies a bit.'
Prime Ministers have feathers (replied true)
'Because in America, the Indians, they live there in America –
    a Prime Minister would be a head man wouldn't he?'
Admirals have fins (replied true)
'Because they go on the ocean where fish are.'
Dragonflies are manufactured goods (replied true)
'They can be.'
Crows are in charge of ships (replied true)
'In the crow's nest.'
Monks have prongs (replied true)
'I thought about their fingernails – prongs, like.'

among the chronically hospitalised populations of mental hospitals, patients who are not grossly intellectually impaired but show a conspicuous deficit in semantic memory. One such example is described in Box 7.2.

Box 7.2 A schizophrenic patient with marked semantic memory impairment

(From McKenna and Laws, 1997)

SR is a 53-year-old woman who became ill in her mid-teenage years and has been chronically hospitalised for the last 20 years. Her presentation is typical of many patients with the most severe and chronic forms of schizophrenia. She is unkempt, with long bedraggled grey hair, and can often be seen wandering around the hospital grounds, sometimes barefoot and in nightclothes, oblivious to the weather. Most of the time she is calm and appears remote with little expression of emotion, but occasionally she has periods lasting days or weeks at a time during which she becomes agitated, paces, and runs up and down corridors, and engages in various destructive behaviours. She has longstanding delusions that her brother is torturing her and that she has the gift of second sight, and she intermittently experiences auditory hallucinations. Much of the time SR's speech is easy to follow but is stilted. She is excessively polite and formal and, when being interviewed thanks all the people in the room after each question. When she is agitated, however, she shows severe thought disorder.

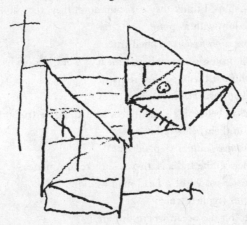

SR is oriented and knows the details of her surroundings, although she is vague when asked about how long she has been in hospital, what wards she has been on, and the names of doctors and nurses who previously looked after her. On neuropsychological testing her score on the Mini-Mental State Examination was 25/30, slightly above the cutoff of 23/24 for mild dementia. Her premorbid IQ, as estimated using the National Adult Reading Test (NART), was 105 and her current WAIS IQ was consistent with this at 93. However she showed a large discrepancy between verbal IQ and performance IQ (106 vs. 76). She performed normally on a number of tests of visual and visuospatial function but was impaired on tasks involving higher levels of perceptual processing, for example identifying objects from silhouettes. As shown, her copying of the Rey Figure was also mildly impaired.

Short-term memory as assessed using span tasks was normal, but she was in the severely impaired range on a number of long-term memory measures. Her executive function was impaired on all tests used. She only achieved 2 out of 6 categories on the modified Wisconsin Card Sorting Test, and scored 17 on the Cognitive Estimates Test, estimating that racehorses gallop at 12 mph and that the length of an average man's spine is 40 feet.

SR was also found to be very impaired on a naming test. She named a kangaroo as a hare, handcuffs as cufflinks, a turtle as a water vole, and an anteater as a beaver. When asked to name the entire corpus of 260 line drawings by Snodgrass and Vanderwart (1980), she made 83 errors, many of which took the form of either semantic category errors (e.g. accordion for trumpet, elephant for rhinoceros) or giving the super-ordinate semantic category rather than the word itself (e.g. musical instrument, vegetable). She also produced some perseverative errors (many animals were named as beaver) and errors based on what seemed to be perceptual confusions (e.g., anchor – 'Cross bones, skull and cross bones'; peanut – 'marrow').

SR was slow on an orally administered version of the 'silly sentences' test but only made two errors, the maximum made by normal subjects. On a slightly harder version of this test (Laws *et al.*, 1995a), however, she made 11 errors out of 56 sentences, well above the upper limit of the normal range of 6. When she was presented with a list made up of 10 high frequency real and 10 non-real words she identified all 20 words as real. She was unable to judge whether words were synonyms at greater than chance levels. Her impairment extended to non-verbal semantic knowledge. The Object Decision Test (Humphreys and Riddoch, 1987) requires subjects to classify drawings of real objects and 'chimeras' (for example, made up by combining the head of one animal with the body of another) as real or imaginary. SR was again barely above chance on this test.

A final area where semantic memory is important is in the recognition of people. To examine this, SR was presented with 53 photographs of famous people and was asked to give their names and as much other identifying information as possible. She managed to name only 9/53 faces and provided the occupations for another six. Most of her other replies consisted of 'don't know' responses, but she also made several stereotyped responses (e.g., Saddam Hussein – 'At a guess, he could be called Lewis'; Clint Eastwood – 'At a guess, he could be called Rupert').

By itself, semantic memory impairment is probably not enough to give rise to thought disorder. This is clear from patients with semantic dementia, where speech is often garrulous, but generally intelligible and may in fact give a superficial impression of normality which conceals the extent of the disorder of vocabulary. Garrard and Hodges (1999) gave the following example of such a patient describing a picture of a soldier:

Oh gosh, this seems to be, oh come on, try to remember the name; I know what they are 'cause there's three of these, so it's not the two and three, it's the one which, er . . . Some of them will be in Britain because, er, you know with our stuff in Britain, some of them are also outside Britain, some of them are also in Britain as well. What d'you call them again because N–'s son, no not son, his brother, he's one of these as well.

However, in schizophrenia, or more precisely in schizophrenic patients with thought disorder, the problem may not be one of permanent loss of information as seen in semantic dementia. Goldberg (Goldberg *et al.*, 1998; Goldberg and Weinberger, 2000) has proposed that there is no large decrement in the amount of information held in semantic memory, but that the organisation of the network is aberrant. In a similar way, Joyce *et al.* (1996) and Laws *et al.* (1998, 1999) have invoked Shallice's (1988) distinction between 'degraded store' and 'impaired access' patterns of semantic memory impairment seen in neurological disorders.[6] The seminal study these authors all cited in this regard was carried out by Allen *et al.* (1993). They gave schizophrenic patients and controls a verbal fluency task and then repeated this four more times. As expected, the patients generated significantly fewer words than the controls. Across the five trials, however, the words they produced varied significantly more. According to Allen *et al.*, this combination of few shared words but many variable words pointed to an inefficient search through a normal-sized word pool, rather than a reduction in the pool of words itself. The tendency to produce variable words was most marked in patients with thought disorder, who also produced more words which were unusual or inappropriate to the category. For example, given the category animals, one patient produced 29 words in three minutes including the following sequence: emu, duck, swan, lake, Loch Ness Monster, bacon, bacon and eggs, pig, porky pig, pig sty (Frith, 1992).

On these grounds, thought disorder should be associated with impairment on some, though not all tests of semantic memory. The best way to demonstrate this is probably not, from the studies of executive function reviewed in the previous

---

[6] Semantic dementia and Alzheimer's disease would be examples of degraded store, whereas a less well-defined group of patients including some with fluent aphasia and others with less clear-cut disorders resulting from temporal lobe lesions show the characteristics of impaired access.

chapter, by means of correlational studies, but by comparing the performance of groups of patients with and without thought disorder, who are preferably intellectually preserved, on a range of different semantic measures. One study fulfils most of these requirements. Goldberg *et al.* (1998) examined a group of twenty-three mainly chronic schizophrenic patients and twenty-three normal controls on four tests probing different aspects of semantic function. The patients and controls were matched for age, although not for estimated premorbid IQ; current IQ was not measured. The patients were dichotomised into those with low ($N = 13$) and high thought disorder scores ($N = 10$) on the basis of ratings on the TLC scale. The semantic memory measures included two tests of knowledge of the meaning of words, the Boston Naming Test and the Peabody Picture Vocabulary Test, where subjects have to indicate which series of four pictures best describes words spoken by the examiner. The third test was the 'silly sentences'. The fourth was a novel measure, semantic fluency minus phonological fluency. In this, the subjects were first to ask to generate as many words in three semantic categories, animals, fruits and vegetables, and then to repeat the exercise with three 'phonological' categories, words beginning with F, A, and S. Fluency tasks are generally considered to require executive function, and so subtracting letter fluency from semantic fluency (the latter typically is larger than the former) can be regarded as testing efficiency of access to knowledge in semantic memory, while controlling for the strategic (i.e. executive) processes necessary to retrieve this information, check it, and monitor it for repetitions, etc. Two executive tests were also given, the Wisconsin Card Sorting Test and letter-number span, a standard test of working memory.

Goldberg *et al.*'s findings are shown in Table 7.4. As expected, the schizophrenic patients showed a pattern of generally poorer performance than the controls. The thought-disordered patients also tended to show lower scores than the non-thought-disordered patients. However, the differences between the two patient groups varied greatly in magnitude across the tests. Performance on the two executive tests did not distinguish the thought-disordered from the non-thought-disordered patients, although the scores on the Wisconsin Card Sorting Test were numerically lower in the former group. Among the semantic tests, naming also failed to distinguish the two patient groups. The thought-disordered patients had lower scores on the word – picture matching task and made nearly twice as many errors on the 'silly sentences' than the controls, but the differences were not significant in either case. However, the measure of semantic minus phonological fluency yielded a marked difference between the thought-disordered and non-thought-disordered patients.

The study of Barrera *et al.* (2004) described in the last chapter replicated some of these findings, in patients who also had relatively intact general intellectual function. Like Goldberg *et al.* (1998) they found no difference in naming performance

Table 7.4 Performance of schizophrenic patients with high and low thought disorder scores on executive and semantic tests

(From Goldberg *et al.*, *American Journal of Psychiatry*, **155,** 1671–1676, Copyright 1998, American Psychiatric Association; http://AJP.psychiatryonline.org. Reprinted by permission)

	Mean score (SD)			
	Normal controls (N = 23)	Mild FTD patients (N = 13)	Moderate/ severe FTD patients (N = 10)	Significant differences
Letter-number span	16.7 (2.5)	13.3 (3.0)	12.7 (4.8)	NC > NFTD and FTD
WCST	8.0 (2.7)	5.7 (3.0)	3.6 (3.6)	NC > FTD
Silly sentences (errors)	1.1 (1.4)	2.2 (2.3)	4.0 (3.7)	NC > NFTD NC > FTD
Peabody Picture Vocabulary	112.2 (13.9)	104.2 (16.0)	95.3 (16.0)	NC > FTD
Boston Naming Test	56.0 (3.2)	55.2 (4.1)	53.6 (3.0)	
Semantic minus phonological fluency	.5.9 (11.8)	8.6 (10.2)	−1.0 (8.0)	NFTD > FTD
Attention test	36.6 (6.0)	36.3 (1.0)	36.3 (1.1)	

between patients with and without thought disorder. Unlike Goldberg *et al.* (1998) they failed to find a difference between the two patient groups on word – picture matching, or on another test requiring judgements about whether words were synonyms or not. The findings with respect to semantic and phonological fluency were in the same direction as those of Goldberg *et al.* – the thought disordered patients were impaired relative to the non-thought disordered patients on semantic fluency and semantic minus phonological fluency, but not on phonological fluency – however, in this study the differences did not reach significance.

Conclusion

The concept of disorganised as opposed to degraded semantic memory brings the dyssemantic hypothesis of thought disorder full circle. In proposing an unstable semantic architecture affecting particularly concepts rather than the meaning of words, authors like Goldberg are returning to a position which is not in the final analysis very different from overinclusive thinking. There is even a touch of irony in such a conclusion. The area of greatest difference in semantic memory performance between the thought-disordered and non-thought-disordered patients in (Barrera *et al*.'s 2004) study was on a further task, the Camel and Cactus Test (Bozeat *et al*., 2000). In this, subjects are shown a series of words, such as *camel*, and they have to decide which of four other words (e.g. tree, sunflower, cactus or rose) it is most closely related to. It is hard to see in what way this differs from the Moran/Epstein test described earlier in this chapter, which was one of the original and most robust tests of overinclusive thinking!

8

Some conclusions and a few speculations

The symptoms of schizophrenia are on the whole anything but subtle, but even so thought disorder stands out from amongst them. There is something about it which arouses curiosity and demands explanation. Part of the reason for this immediacy may be, as the psychologist Harvey has pointed out, that it is one of the few signs in psychiatry – an objectively observable abnormality as opposed to a subjective description of some aspect of one's inner mental state. But whatever it is, a great deal of ink has been spilled by psychiatrists trying to describe and psychologists trying to explain just what it is that makes the patient difficult to follow.

Unfortunately the answer to these questions appears to be 'more than one thing'. The price of describing thought disorder reliably has been the acceptance of a large and unwieldy set of abnormalities, and this book has only narrowly avoided finding support for every theory ever proposed to explain it. In such circumstances integrative models are customarily reached for. For integrative one can usually read complicated, and the term model conjures up something which is not testable and accompanied by flow diagrams. Without resorting to models, and resisting any temptation to inflict flow diagrams on the reader, what follows offers some not very systematic suggestions on how the different elements of thought disorder and their underpinnings might be reduced to something more manageable.

Why is thought disorder so complicated?

At the clinical level the main issue confronting thought disorder is not, as Rochester and Martin thought, its circularity but its complexity. There seems to be no way of avoiding the unwelcome conclusion that thought disorder comprises a number of quite different abnormalities which combine and recombine erratically, often in the same patient. When thought-disordered patients are rated using the TLC scale, they almost always score on a variety of items. As demonstrated in the examples scattered throughout this book, even patients whose predominant abnormality is derailment, poverty of content or stiltedness can generally be relied on to also show one or two word approximations, neologisms or clang associations.

This is an untidy, even embarrassing position to be in. A lot of time and effort has been devoted to pursuing some common thread in the features of thought disorder which, as with the proverbial blind men feeling the elephant, would make sense of all of them. These efforts began with Kraepelin (1913a) who proposed that the process of derailment could be applied not just to the train of thought, but also to the construction of sentences, leading to what he called akataphasia, and to the selection of words themselves, resulting in neologisms. Orders of magnitude more influential was Bleuler's (1911) attempt to subsume all aspects of thought disorder under the general heading of loose associations, which Rochester and Martin (1979) were probably right to attack. The theory behind it was certainly vague, perhaps tautological and, most damning of all, ultimately sterile.

The different elements of thought disorder may not be manifestations of a single symptom, but they certainly tend to run together. As described in Chapter 2, there is plenty of empirical support for the status of thought disorder as a syndrome. Derailment, tangentiality, loss of goal and incoherence form a highly intercorrelated core cluster of abnormalities which provide the basis for the clinical stereotype of thought-disordered speech. Illogicality, circumstantiality, and pressure of speech seem to be a more variable part of the same cluster. Even poverty of content of speech, considered by Andreasen, to be part of a separate syndrome of negative thought disorder, has been found to show positive correlations with these items in some correlational and factor analytic studies – including her own.

The fact that thought disorder has many clinical features but that most of these are related to each other obviously needs to be reconciled. One possible way of doing so is by invoking the continuum of severity of thought disorder introduced in Chapter 2. On this argument, what is referred to as poverty of content of speech is the mildest expression of a process which disorganises thought; as this becomes more severe, clearly identifiable instances of derailment and loss of goal appear; ultimately speech is affected to such a degree that it disrupts individual sentences and is called incoherence. If so, it could also be that as the disturbance worsens it becomes not only deeper but broader – an initially unitary disturbance progressively draws in other abnormalities, or allows them to escape from check. A more mechanistic way of conceptualising the same idea is that a low grade breakdown in, say, the cognitive machinery that converts thought into speech will affect only one particular component of this. However, as disorder increases, the capacity of the rest of the system is strained and errors in other parts of the process begin to creep in.

Thought disorder outside schizophrenia

Outside of the inward-looking and deeply psychoanalytically influenced movement that enveloped American psychiatry for several decades, no-one seriously believed that thought disorder was only seen in schizophrenia. For one thing, it has always been all too evident in mania for this. Once psychoanalysis relaxed its grip and American psychiatrists were allowed to observe rather than interpret, no time was lost in asking questions about the occurrence of the phenomenon in other disorders as well, from depression to epilepsy to autism.

Since it is clear from Chapter 3 that disorder of the form of thinking is a quite widespread clinical phenomenon, the question becomes not whether it occurs but how much its pattern varies from disorder to disorder. It would be convenient if thought disorder in each different condition was characterised by a unique set of abnormalities – poverty of content, derailment, tangentiality, neologisms, etc. in schizophrenia; distractibility and pressure of speech in mania; circumstantiality in epilepsy; and so on. Unfortunately, the most that can probably be said is that different disorders may show a different profile of high and low TLC scores, but that patients with any disorder can score on all TLC items. A case can be made that schizophrenic and manic forms of thought disorder each have their own distinctive stamp, but Andreasen's work has shown that the distinction is a slightly tenuous one, and the similarities outweigh the differences. The thought disorder of psychosis shows little overlap with that seen in autism and epilepsy, but whether it differs in these latter two disorders is a moot point. There has been a curious reluctance to call the incoherent speech seen in delirium thought disorder, but would edited transcripts of incoherent delirious patients be identified under blind conditions as different from those of thought-disordered schizophrenic or manic patients? It is not clear that anyone would take the bet.

Discussions of thought disorder outside schizophrenia often start with a declaration that it can occur in normal subjects and finish with speculation about its possible relationship to creativity. The former statement can be regarded as reasonably well established, although the evidence base is somewhere between small and tiny. The latter statement depends mainly on a larger but equally amorphous literature on the link between madness and creativity. Some authors, for example those cited in Chapter 3, have argued that the association is with schizophrenia. Jamison (1993) has effectively championed the view that the real association is with mania. Nettle (2001) has mounted a detailed argument that both disorders are associated with creativity in different ways, but that this is not expressed in the vast majority of patients. Thought disorder is usually a port of call in these accounts, but it never forms the main thrust of the argument. But perhaps thought disorder *is* the important link – the similarity between the writings of Joyce and schizophrenic thought disorder, and the effortless witty and novel productions of manic patients are both remarkable – and an obvious test of this hypothesis would be if there were further links with creativity in the other disorders where the symptom is seen.

One disorder where such a case can be made is autism. It used to be thought that individuals with the high functioning form of this disorder and those with Asperger's syndrome were lacking in normal creativity, a view which is enshrined in DSM IV and ICD-10. This is despite the fact that Asperger (1944), in his original account, stated that some patients showed particular originality of thought and experience, which could lead to exceptional achievements in later life. It is now being belatedly recognised that several of the most brilliant achievements in human history have been made by individuals who showed unmistakeable evidence of being autistic. These predictably include a number of mathematicians and scientists, including Newton (definitely) and Einstein (possibly) among others (James, 2003). Fitzgerald (2004) has also argued that the list should be extended to a philosopher, Wittgenstein, a writer, Lewis Carroll, a poet, Yeats, and perhaps even certain politicians.

The link with creativity also unexpectedly surfaces in another group of individuals who may show a form of thought disorder, eccentrics. Weeks and James (1995) concluded that the 1,000 plus eccentrics they interviewed had a number of traits in common, which were as far flung as being of above-average intelligence, having unusual eating habits and being a bad speller. Five characteristics, however, could be seen in virtually every eccentric. In approximate descending order of frequency, these were: non-conforming, creative, strongly motivated by curiosity, idealistic and happily obsessed with one or more hobbyhorses. They went on to state:

Creativity is at the heart of eccentricity. One of the principal reasons eccentrics continually challenge the established order is because they want to experiment, to try out new ways of doing things. That quality is most conspicuous in artists and scientists, who are significantly more likely to be eccentric than the rest of us. The study included 75 artists, whose lives are, obviously, devoted to creative activity, as well as many inventors, who use their brainpower to bring into existence entirely new and presumably useful machines. But some of our eccentrics were driven, it seems, not by traditional aesthetic or scientific impulses but rather by a powerful need to create in its purest, generalized form. One such person is John Ward, of Northamptonshire, who describes himself as a junkist. He constructs fantastical machines from other people's rubbish. On the day the Prince and Princess of Wales got married, he celebrated by welding together three bathtubs to make a catamaran for his four children.

Thought disorder: a disorder of thought, language or both?

Rochester and Martin (1979) were critical of Bleuler and those who followed him for propagating the view that thought disorder was a disorder of thought rather than language. Possibly they overstated this criticism – the only subsequent authors to claim categorically that there is no abnormality of language in schizophrenia have been a handful of neurologists who perhaps should have known better than to pontificate on the issue. In another sense, though, Rochester and Martin were on the mark: there was and to some extent still is a suffocating orthodoxy which prevents language being discussed in relation to thought disorder – except as hedged around with so many qualifications and reservations it no longer deserves the designation of language. What this has always been about is distancing thought disorder from dysphasia, with all that this would imply for the status of schizophrenia as a psychiatric as opposed to a neurological disease.

Where there is an established order, there will always be a heretic to challenge it. Kleist (1960) threw down the gauntlet for the neurological view of thought disorder in the boldest possible terms when he stated, complete with italics: 'We are therefore dealing with *sensory aphasic impairments* similar to those found in focal brain lesions of the *left temporal lobe*.' But it was another, if anything more outspoken author, Chaika, who started the process which led to Kleist's eventual vindication – the evidence from her studies, plus the others reviewed in Chapter 4, places the existence of genuinely linguistic abnormalities in thought disorder beyond reasonable doubt.

Why this should be so is a mystery, one which is probably part of the larger mystery of why thought disorder is a multiplex disorder in the first place. Part of the solution may be contained in what Kleist (1960) qualified the above statement with:

The only difference is the involvement in schizophrenia of higher levels of speech which are responsible for word derivations, word constructions, the formation of sentences, and for the abstract meaning of speech conceptions – i.e. the thinking based on speech. On the other hand in focal brain lesions the lower levels of speech, i.e. the sounds, words (sound sequences) and names are disturbed.

He then went on to claim that disorders of speech-based thought could be detected in patients with focal neurological lesions from war wounds. Is it possible, perhaps, that all the time that psychiatry was doing its best to ignore Kleist and others who pointed to linguistic abnormality in thought disorder, neurology was just as studiously looking the other way concerning the occurrence of features which are customarily the preserve of psychiatry in patients with dysphasia? Consider the following account by Weinstein *et al.* (1981) describing patients with jargon aphasia:

Jargon patients also seek to give the impression of being erudite. They use a greater proportion of low frequency words than do standard aphasics and their speech contains ornate phraseology, pedantic redundancies, and 'high sounding' malapropisms. When one patient was asked what was wrong with him, he replied with *Well, it has been suggested that there were certain oddities and restrictions, technically the activities of the student body, so to speak.* Even when speech has improved and the patient no longer has neologisms, he tends to make unusual word choices. For example, one man commented on the *congestion* of his speech, and another recalled having done a lot of *verbal gambling* with words. When tested for ability to generate rhymes, alliterations, synonyms, antonyms, and homonyms, patients produce strings of impressive sounding but inappropriate words. A woman 'rhymed' the following: *Ovoid, ovum, spectrum, parallax, quadrangle, trigonometry, algebra.* Some subjects speak officialese. The use of alliterations and assonances and an exaggerated rhythm may impart a poetic quality.

When the boundary between two classes of symptoms seems to be blurred, when similar phenomena with different names crop up in both, and when their identity or otherwise is a matter of inconclusive debate, the time may have come to entertain the biggest heresy of all: Rogers' (1985; 1992) 'conflict of paradigms' hypothesis. He (see Box 8.1) investigated the kinds of motor disorder shown by chronically hospitalised schizophrenic patients, which is conventionally believed to take two forms. On the one hand there are the neurological side effects of neuroleptic drugs, the extrapyramidal symptoms of parkinsonism and tardive dyskinesia. On the other are the catatonic symptoms of schizophrenia, which include some simple disorders of movement, such as stereotypies, mannerisms, waxy flexibility, along with more complex phenomena like stupor, excitement, negativism and automatic obedience. When Rogers examined the patients, however, what he found did not fall neatly into two categories; instead, he was confronted by a mass of abnormalities, which certainly spanned a range from simple to very complex but which it was futile to try and disentangle from one another.

Box 8.1 The motor disorders of severe psychiatric illness: a conflict of paradigms

(From Rogers, 1985)

Rogers examined motor disorder in a group of 100 patients on the long stay wards of a mental hospital. Almost all of these had been given a diagnosis of schizophrenia at some point. He assessed abnormalities in a non-prejudicial way, avoiding use of terms which pre-empted their designation as neurological or psychiatric. Abnormalities were simply classified under headings of posture, tone, purposive movement, activity, abnormal movements, etc.

All the patients showed some evidence of motor disorder. This included *disorder of posture and tone*, characteristically a tendency to flexion associated with varying degrees of rigidity and typically affecting the head and neck; *disorder of motor performance*, both spontaneous and elicited, characteristically difficulty with the initiation, efficient execution of, or persistence with purposive motor activity;

Box 8.1 (cont.)

disorder of motor activity, characteristically inappropriate activity, ranging from the short-lived, spontaneous and violent to the continual, stimulus-dependent and quasi-purposeful; *abnormal movements*, ranging from the random, simple and abrupt to the regular, complex and co-ordinated; *disorder of automatic movements*, such as walking and blinking; and *disorder of speech production*, with abnormalities reflecting those of the motor system generally. These abnormalites ranged from the simple to very complex, and in-between were all sorts of intermediate forms which could not easily be categorised as either neurological (i.e. extrapyramidal) or psychiatric (i.e. catatonic).

The pattern was similar in all respects when Rogers rated motor disorder recorded in the patients' case notes before 1955, the year antipsychotic drugs began to be used in the hospital. In particular there was roughly the same amount of simple dyskinesia-like movements and parkinsonism-like slowness.

Rogers' conclusion was that there was a 'conflict of paradigms', with neurological and psychiatric schools of thought both attempting to describe what were in reality a broad set of phenomena which transcended both disciplines. He illustrated his argument with the two pictures shown below. The one on the left, from a 1928 psychiatric textbook, was titled grimacing mannerism in dementia praecox. The one on the right is from Kinnear Wilson's neurological textbook of the same era and shows a mandibular tic in a patient with post-encephalitic parkinsonism. Two different vocabularies were being used to describe what were on the face of it the same phenomenon.

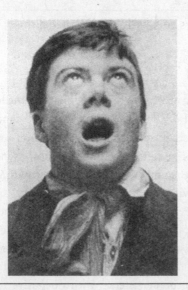 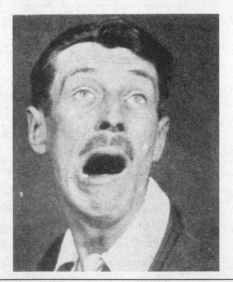

Rogers' radical interpretation was that two different conceptual frameworks had grown up to describe parts of what was in reality a continuously varying spectrum of abnormality. This was ultimately a consequence of the historical divergence between neurology and psychiatry at the turn of the twentieth century, which was in turn mainly due to the influence of psychoanalysis on the latter discipline. Could it be that there is a similar conflict of paradigms between neurological and psychiatric speech disorders? That they too can both only be properly understood as different points on a neuropsychiatric continuum?

Thought disorder as a non-dysphasic language disturbance

Whether or not Rogers' perspective is the right way to look at thought disorder, there is no getting away from the fact there is more to schizophrenic speech than dysphasia. Dysphasia-like abnormalities make up only a small proportion of the abnormality of thought disorder, which is in fact quite easy to overlook among its other manifestations; the speech of Chaika's (1974) patient described in Chapter 4 is not obviously similar to that of a dysphasic patient. One way of increasing the power of a linguistic theory of thought disorder is by broadening it to include higher levels of speech, which Kleist somewhat vaguely referred to as the abstract meaning of speech conceptions and the thinking based on speech, but which can now be specified more precisely as communicative competence.

The first foray into this field was Rochester and Martin's (1979) proposal that thought-disordered schizophrenic speakers fail to employ cohesive ties to the same extent as normal individuals, and it promptly had negative results: although schizophrenic patients used significantly fewer cohesive ties than normal speakers, there was no difference between those with and without thought disorder. What did characterise thought-disordered speech in Rochester and Martin's study was the abnormal use of one class of tie, that of reference. This latter finding has been replicated, if not always particularly transparently, in several further studies, with that of Oh *et al.* (2002) suggesting that it is part of a broader abnormality in semantics at the level of discourse. However, it is clear from this last study that the contribution of erroneous use of ties to thought disorder is once again small.

Chapman and Chapman's (1973) and Kuperberg *et al.*'s (1998) lack of use of linguistic context can expand the role for higher-order language abnormalities in thought disorder further, as well as continuing the theme of semantic abnormality. However, abnormality in another 'higher-order' area of language, pragmatics, emerges with no real support. The idea that thought disorder stems from an ability to take into account the listener's needs, which owes much to the theoretical work of Frith (1992), is intuitively appealing. But ironically, these studies, some of the most ingenious of which were also carried out by Frith, have not managed to find associations with thought disorder, although correlations with other symptoms have otherwise been easy to demonstrate.

Surely, one might argue, it is premature to exclude a pragmatic deficit in thought disorder – more studies are needed, or the existing ones have focused on the wrong aspects of theory of mind; perhaps a meta-analysis would provide more solid support. But there is a good reason to accept the findings at face value. This is because we already have an excellent clinical model for the effect of a theory of mind or pragmatic deficit on speech, but this is autism, not schizophrenia. As Chapter 3 makes clear, the points of correspondence between the speech disorder of autism and Asperger's syndrome and schizophrenic thought disorder are not very great.

Beyond language

No matter how broadly defined, it seems likely that language is only ever going to be able to account for a limited amount of the abnormality underlying thought disorder. Even a hardened advocate of the neurological approach to schizophrenia like Kleist (1930) conceded that not all the disordered speech in schizophrenics originates from an aphasia-like language disorder. Needless to say, he was confident that at least some of the additional disorders of thinking would be explicable in organic terms. While the search for these factors has covered a lot of ground, the two that have survived are, as Kleist predicted, either wholly or partly neuropsychological in nature.

McGrath gave the frontal lobes considerable power to explain certain features of thought disorder, and Liddle initiated a series of studies which have implicated executive impairment in the disorganisation syndrome. There are, it is true, a number of caveats and qualifications to this conclusion. One which immediately presents itself is that executive impairment is at least as strongly associated with negative symptoms as with disorganisation. Another difficulty for the frontal/dysexecutive theory of thought disorder is that, while there is good evidence that frontal lobe lesions can give rise to incoherent speech, this seems to be a rather pale imitation of thought disorder as seen in schizophrenia.

In the simple neuropsychological sense, a semantic memory account of thought disorder faces similar difficulties. The speech of patients with semantic dementia is abnormal, but not in a way which resembles that of thought-disordered schizophrenic patients. A related and even bigger problem is that patients with semantic dementia have above all a loss of knowledge of the meaning of words. However, while impaired naming is certainly part of the pattern of the cognitive impairment seen in schizophrenia, and can sometimes be quite severe (e.g. Laws *et al.*, 2000), virtually every study that has been done has found that naming performance does not distinguish patients with and without thought disorder. The concept of disorganised rather than degraded semantic memory might be able to get round this difficulty to some extent, but the body of evidence on this point is small and the findings are not especially consistent.

The fact that both of the two main psychological approaches to thought disorder seem inadequate may not be a problem but an opportunity. This is because thought disorder is itself not a unitary clinical phenomenon. If any attempt to reduce the different elements of thought disorder to a single phenomenon is doomed to failure, then there is no reason to expect a single cognitive abnormality to reproduce it in all respects – in some ways this is the last thing that is wanted. It then becomes possible to envisage that a dysexecutive impairment giving rise to 'frontal lobe' speech, which strays from its theme, is careless and replete with word play, embellishments and so on, might interact with something akin to the empty speech of semantic dementia, producing a result that is different to that seen in each of the disorders individually.

There might even be a precedent for this in the neurological literature. The presentations of fronto-temporal dementia are commonly not pure, and patients often show combinations of frontal lobe and temporal lobe features, particularly as the disease progresses. Snowden *et al.* (1996) described one such case, a sixty-nine-year-old retired headmaster and mathematician. He showed a speech disorder characterised by fluent, pressured speech, which was irrelevant and disconnected. He switched between topics and juxtaposed elements inappropriately. Objects his gaze momentarily rested on and words in the interviewer's questions would be repeated and incorporated into what he was saying. His speech was syntactically correct, and apart from some stereotyped use of words (e.g. 'system'), there were few paraphasic errors. Word comprehension and naming, although not normal, were substantially better than expected. At post-mortem he was found to have severe atrophy of the temporal lobes, which was bilateral but more marked on the right, plus more symmetrical mild to moderate atrophy in the frontal lobes. An example of his speech[1] is shown in Box 8.2. It is a reasonable facsimile of poverty of content of speech, and at a number of points the patient also slips away from the point of the question.

---

[1] This is not published but was kindly provided by Dr J. S. Snowden.

Box 8.2 The speech of LP, a patient with fronto-temporal dementia showing mixed language and behavioural disorder

(From Snowden *et al.*, 1996)

Q   Tell me about your job then.

A   Ah well the jobs are very interesting, I like these things. We have got a very big car, it is an SRI and it is a very powerful thing that one and we got it in there at the time and I had a very, very good piece of work. My wife now goes even faster on that than she can by herself, do you see. The other ones there we have got all sorts of people who have got great and interesting ideas with us. We have got lots and lots of our people coming in, do you see, and we get it in there at that time and we have two or three friends there and a friend there and another one here and another one there and another one there all the way round, do you see, and that's what's going to be coming for the next few days, do you see, and my wife of course, she disappeared, now I don't know where she went to. There was a case there where it was about I suppose really um it must have been quite easy altogether for them, they could have put . . . . I have got a very nice house in this one and it was very easy to have all these items and it was something like this sort of size but of course we had all sorts of lovely things and a dear little girl here, a tiny little girl about this size who could speak, run about and everything at all, she is only about three years old. She is a very attractive little thing, beautiful little thing, she is marvellous. Then some of the others come through there and also I have myself a which is in this area and that's the area for the whole of the question here for Stockport.

Q   A railcard.

A   That will be for one year that I have got for the whole system.

Q   So you can travel around.

A   Yes that's from Euston. From Euston it is a tremendous amount going onto it. It's a huge area and we have got them now, do you see. Well it is really very interesting if you like to have these ideas. But of course in other parts of it the electricity ones are really very, very able and they come on all the place all the time.

Q   Can you tell me about your job as a headmaster?

A   As a head. As a headmaster. Oh, I had a big one. I had around 3000 boys I think I heard about it. They were very good indeed – and this was a bit of a tragedy of my own stupidity – and it really was so awful, I discovered afterwards. What happened was that eventually I could have, I decided that I wanted to have enough after I had done a whole lot of these things which were very difficult, there were some very nasty children there and I thought

> well this seems to be getting rather ridiculous and also particularly serious –
> one boy had been killed, they stuck a knife into him, do you see. A very serious
> matter indeed and I thought well, if it is going to do that sort of system I shall
> probably decide to hold part of this part and he would be able possibly to do
> something about it. I then went to see the biggest man there of the area. The
> whole system of these went right the way across, and I went to see him and he
> said, yes well what you can do to stop this is, you can have the whole lot put on
> and you can have a special amount of money for whatever you like and you can
> get the whole lot. And I got about £6000 or so for them, anything like that you
> see and that was the idea. After that I thought, Oh this is marvellous, now I had
> things called calculus, you may not have heard of calculus have you?

This speech, however, still lacks some of the qualities of thought-disordered
schizophrenic speech. The similarity to schizophrenic thought disorder might be
closer if the semantic memory abnormality was one of disorganisation rather than
a loss in the amount of information. Just what additional qualities increased
semantic priming would also bring is unclear, but it could only add to the richness
of the abnormality.

Thought disorder: semantic confabulation?

As noted in passing in Chapter 6, frontal/executive impairment is associated with
one further unusual clinical phenomenon in neurological patients. This is confabulation, the tendency to volunteer invented information when asked questions,
usually about personal events. Confabulation itself does not resemble thought
disorder; Baddeley and Wilson's (1986, 1988) patient gave an essentially lucid
account of facts which were untrue and events which never happened. However,
since leading current theories explain the phenomenon as an abnormal interaction
between executive function and memory, it may be worth seeing if there is any
scope for adapting the model to account for some aspects of thought disorder.

According to Baddeley (1990), recollection is a demanding task involving
checking and reconstruction. This is likely to be even more difficult in the presence
of amnesia, and, if such patients also have a deficit in executive function, they may
'in the difficult task of filtering out truth from invention, opt for the easy invention
rather than the hazy and difficult truth'. In the most detailed articulation of the
dysexecutive hypothesis of confabulation, Moscovitch (1989, 1995; Moscovitch
and Melo, 1997) has argued that confabulation is related to a distinction between
two well-accepted processes that take place during memory retrieval, associative
and strategic. Associative or cue dependent retrieval is a relatively automatic
process, in which a cue interacts automatically and mandatorily with information

stored in memory, a process termed 'ecphory'. The product is either the memory that is sought or some other memory that serves as material for further searches. Strategic retrieval processes, on the other hand, are conscious, effortful, problem-solving routines that are brought into play when the associative process is ineffective. They are involved in initiating and organising a search to locate a cue that allows the associative process to deliver the right solution. Once the memory is recovered, these processes then evaluate and verify the accuracy of the recovered memory and place it in its proper temporal–spatial context. Confabulation occurs when there is damage to strategic retrieval processes that leads to defective search, poor monitoring or faulty output from memory, and leaves recollection overly dependent on automatic associative processes. In the words of Moscovitch (1989), the confabulating patient:

haphazardly combines information from disparate events, jumbles their sequence, and essentially accepts as veridical whatever the ecphoric process delivers to consciousness. The minimal organization that his memories show is dependent on the loose rules of plausibility and association rather than on systematic strategies aimed at recovering additional ecphoric information. In cases of fantastic confabulation, retrieval information interacts with whatever information is currently active in the perceptual and semantic modules to deliver ecphoric information that reflects recent thoughts, perceptions or fantasies rather than relevant past experiences.

If the same abnormal processes were to also take place in semantic memory, and semantic confabulation is known to occur (e.g. Laws *et al.*, 1995b); if the term ecphory were to be replaced by spreading activation, which Tulving (1985) appears to believe it can; and if the defective strategic processes had to contend not only with impairment, but also with disorganisation or even an increased ecphory due to hyperpriming, might not thought disorder be the plausible result?

This proposal has the merit that it might be able to explain illogicality. This can be defined without difficulty as the uncritical acceptance that there is a relationship between two propositions when in fact there is none. Or, using the above terminology, the conscious experience of echory which occurs when the spread of activation from two nodes in semantic memory intersects is accepted without any further checks and reconstruction. Thus, when asked the question from a test designed to elicit confabulation, 'What is the main diet of the duck-billed platypus?', a thought-disordered schizophrenic patient replied 'eggs'[2] – for him, the mere existence of link between platypus and eggs was enough to verify the proposition implied in the question. The same process could be construed as taking place in the example of illogicality Andreasen (1979a) used in the TLC scale:

---

[2] The correct answer is worms, shellfish and grubs.

Parents are the people that raise you. Anything that raises you can be a parent. Parents can be anything, material, vegetable, or mineral, that has taught you something. Parents would be the world of things that are alive, that are there. Rocks, a person can look at a rock and learn something from it, so that would be a parent.

There may even be examples of thought disorder which contain the actual violations of knowledge about the world usually implied by the term semantic confabulation. Consider this extract of the speech of Chaika's (1974) patient described in Chapter 4, which is liberally peppered with what by any standard would have to be called semantic confabulations:

My mother's name was Bill. (pause) (low pitch, as in an aside, but with marked rising question intonation) ... and coo? St. Valentine's Day is the official startin' of the breedin' season of the birds. All buzzards can coo. I like to see it pronounced buzzards rightly. They work hard. So do parakeets.

The authors have not been able to confirm that all of the unlikely propositions in this passage of speech are in fact false, but they certainly conflict with information in their semantic memories.

References

Studies included in the meta-analysis in Chapter 7 are marked with an asterisk.

Alexander, M.P., Benson, D.F. and Stuss, D.T. (1989). Frontal lobes and language. *Brain and Language*, **37**, 656–691.

Allen, H.A., Liddle, P.F. and Frith, C.D. (1993). Negative features, retrieval processes and verbal fluency in schizophrenia. *British Journal of Psychiatry*, **163**, 769–775.

*Aloia, M.S., Gourovitch, M.L., Missar, D., Pickar, D., Weinberger, D.R. and Goldberg, T.E. (1998). Cognitive substrates of thought disorder, II: specifying a candidate cognitive mechanism. *American Journal of Psychiatry*, **155**, 1677–1684.

Andreasen, N.C. (1979a). Thought, language and communication disorders: I. Clinical assessment, definition of terms and evaluation of their reliability. *Archives of General Psychiatry*, **36**, 1315–1321.

(1979b). Affective flattening and the criteria for schizophrenia. *American Journal of Psychiatry*, **136**, 944–947.

(1979c). Thought, language, and communication disorders: II. Diagnostic significance. *Archives of General Psychiatry*, **36**, 1325–1330.

(1982). Negative symptoms in schizophrenia: definition and reliability. *Archives of General Psychiatry*, **39**, 784–788.

(1987). *The Comprehensive Assessment of Symptoms and History*. Iowa city: University of Iowa College of Medicine.

Andreasen, N.C., Arndt, S., Alliger, R., Miller, D. and Flaum, M. (1995). Symptoms of schizophrenia: methods, meanings, and mechanisms. *Archives of General Psychiatry*, **52**, 341–351.

Andreasen, N.C. and Grove, W.M. (1986a). Evaluation of positive and negative symptoms in schizophrenia. *Psychiatrie et Psychobiologie*, **1**, 108–121.

(1986b). Thought, language, and communication in schizophrenia: diagnosis and prognosis. *Schizophrenia Bulletin*, **12**, 348–359.

Andreasen, N.C. and Olsen, S. (1982). Negative v. positive schizophrenia: definition and validation. *Archives of General Psychiatry*, **39**, 789–794.

Andreasen, N.J.C. and Powers, P.S. (1974). Overinclusive thinking in mania and schizophrenia. *British Journal of Psychiatry*, **125**, 452–456.

Andreasen, N.J.C., Tsuang, M.T. and Canter, A. (1974). The significance of thought disorder in diagnostic evaluations. *Comprehensive Psychiatry*, **15**, 27–34.

Arnold, A. (1969). *James Joyce*. New York: Frederick Ungar.

Arora, A., Avasthi, A. and Kulhara, P. (1997). Subsyndromes of chronic schizophrenia: a phenomenological study. *Acta Psychiatrica Scandinavica*, **96**, 225–229.

Asperger, H. (1944). Die 'Autistic Psychopathen' im Kindeshalter. *Archiv fur Psychiatrie und Nervenkrankheiten*, **117**, 76–136. [Translated by U. Frith (1991) as 'Autistic Psychopathy' in childhood. In *Autism and Asperger Syndrome*, ed. U. Frith. Cambridge: Cambridge University Press.]

Astrup, C. (1979). *The Chronic Schizophrenias*. Oslo: Universitetsforlaget.

Baddeley, A. (1986). *Working Memory*. Oxford: Oxford University Press.

(1990). *Human Memory: Theory and Practice*. Hove: Erlbaum.

(1996). Exploring the central executive. *Quarterly Journal of Experimental Psychology*, **49A**, 5–28.

Baddeley, A. and Wilson, B. (1986). Amnesia, autobiographical memory and confabulation. In *Autobiographical Memory*, ed. D.C. Rubin. Cambridge: Cambridge University Press.

(1988). Frontal amnesia and the dysexecutive syndrome. *Brain and Cognition*, **7**, 212–230.

Barber, F., Pantelis, C., Bodger, S. and Nelson, H. (1996). Intellectual functioning in schizophrenia: natural history. In *Schizophrenia: A Neuropsychological Perspective*, ed. C. Pantelis, H.E. Nelson and T.R.E. Barnes. Chicester: Wiley.

*Barch, D.M., Carter, C.S., Perlstein, W., Baird, J., Cohen, J.D. and Schooler, N. (1999). Increased stroop facilitation effects in schizophrenia are not due to increased automatic semantic priming. *Schizophrenia Research*, **39**, 51–64.

*Barch, D.M., Cohen, J.D., Servan-Schreiber, D., Steingard, S., Cohen, J.D., Steinhauer, S.S. and van Kammen, D.P. (1996). Semantic priming in schizophrenia: an examination of spreading activation using word pronunciation and multiple SOAs. *Journal of Abnormal Psychology*, **105**, 592–601.

Barrera, A., McKenna, P.J. and Berrios, G.E. (2004). Formal thought disorder in schizophrenia: an executive or a semantic deficit? *Psychological Medicine*, in press.

Basso, M.R., Nasrallah, H.A., Olson, S.C. and Bornstein, R.A. (1998). Neuropsychological correlates of negative, disorganized and psychotic symptoms in schizophrenia. *Schizophrenia Research*, **31**, 99–111.

*Baving, L., Wagner, M., Cohen, R. and Rockstroh, B. (2001). Increased semantic and repetition priming in schizophrenic patients. *Journal of Abnormal Psychology*, **110**, 67–75.

Baxter, R.D. and Liddle, P.F. (1998). Neuropsychological deficits associated with schizophrenic syndromes. *Schizophrenia Research*, **30**, 239–249.

Bear, D.M. (1979). Temporal lobe epilepsy: a syndrome of sensory-limbic hyperconnection. *Cortex*, **15**, 357–384.

Bear, D.M. and Fedio, P. (1977). Quantitative analysis of interictal behavior in temporal lobe epilepsy. *Archives of Neurology*, **34**, 454–467.

Bear, D., Levin, K., Blumer, D., Chetham, D. and Ryder, J. (1982). Interictal behaviour in hospitalised temporal lobe epileptics: relationship to idiopathic psychiatric syndromes. *Journal of Neurology, Neurosurgery and Psychiatry*, **45**, 481–488.

Bell, M.D., Lysaker, P.H., Milstein, R.M. and Beam-Goulet, J.L. (1994). Concurrent validity of the cognitive component of schizophrenia: relationship of PANSS scores to neuropsychological assessments. *Psychiatry Research*, **54**, 51–58.

Benjamin, T.B. and Watt, T.F. (1969). Psychopathology and semantic interpretation of ambiguous words. *Journal of Abnormal Psychology*, **74**, 706–714.

Benson, D.F. (1973). Psychiatric aspects of aphasia. *British Journal of Psychiatry*, **123**, 555–566.

Berrios, G.E. (1985). Positive and negative symptoms and Jackson. *Archives of General Psychiatry*, **42**, 95–97.

(1991). Positive and negative signals: a conceptual history. In *Negative Versus Positive Schizophrenia*, ed. A. Marneros, N.C. Andreasen and M.T. Tsuang. Berlin/Heidelberg: Springer Verlag.

*Besche-Richard, C. and Passerieux, C. (2003). Semantic context-processing deficit in thought-disordered schizophrenic patients: evidence from new semantic priming paradigms. *Cognitive Neuropsychiatry*, **8**, 173–189.

*Besche, C., Passerieux, C., Segui, J., Sarfati, Y., Laurent, J.-P. and Hardy-Bayle, M.C. (1997). Syntactic and semantic processing in schizophrenic patients evaluated by lexical-decision tasks. *Neuropsychology*, **11**, 498–505.

Bilder, R.M., Mukherjee, S., Rieder, R.O. and Pandurangi, A.K. (1985). Symptomatic and neuropsychological components of defect states. *Schizophrenia Bulletin*, **11**, 409–419.

Bishop, D.V.M. (1989). *Test for the Reception of Grammar*, 2nd edn. London: Medical Research Council.

(1997). *Uncommon Understanding: Development and Disorders of Language Comprehension in Children*. Hove: Psychology Press.

(2000). Pragmatic language impairment: a correlate of SLI, a distinct subgroup, or part of the autistic continuum. In *Speech and Language Impairments in Children: Causes, Characteristics, Intervention and Outcome*, ed. D.V.M. Bishop and L.B. Leonard. Hove: Psychology Press.

Bishop, D.V.M. and Rosenbloom, L. (1987). Classification of childhood language disorders. In *Language Development and Disorders: Clinics in Developmental Medicine* (Double Issue), ed. W. Yale and M. Rutter. London: MacKeith Press.

Bishop, D.V.M. and Adams, C. (1989). Conversational characteristics of children with semantic-pragmatic disorder. II. What features lead to a judgement of inappropriacy? *British Journal of Disorders of Communication*, **24**, 241–263.

Blakey, A.F., Hellewell, J.S.E. and Deakin, J.F.W. (1996). Thought disorder in schizophrenia reflects general cognitive impairment and not focal linguistic dysfunction. *Schizophrenia Research*, **18**, 205.

Blaney, T. (1974). Two studies on the language behaviour in schizophrenics. *Journal of Abnormal Psychology*, **83**: 23–31.

Blashfield, R.K. (1984). *The Classification of Psychopathology: Neo-Kraepelinian and Quantitative Approaches*. New York: Plenum Press.

Bleuler, E. (1911) *Dementia Praecox or the Group of Schizophrenias* (trans. J. Zinkin, 1950). New York: International Universities Press.

*Blum, N.A. and Freides, D. (1995). Investigating thought disorder in schizophrenia with the lexical decision task. *Schizophrenia Research*, **16**, 217–224.

Blumer, D. (1975). Temporal lobe epilepsy and its psychiatric significance. In *Psychiatric Aspects of Neurologic Disease*, ed. D.F. Benson and D. Blumer. New York: Grune & Stratton.

(1995). Personality disorders in epilepsy. In *Neuropsychiatry of Personality Disorders*, ed. J.J. Ratey. Oxford: Blackwell Science.

Blumer, D. and Benson, D.F. (1975). Personality changes with frontal and temporal lobe lesions. In *Psychiatric Aspects of Neurological Disease*, ed. D.F. Benson and D. Blumer. New York: Grune & Stratton.

(1982). Psychiatric manifestations of epilepsy. In *Psychiatric Aspects of Neurological Disease*, Vol II, ed. D.F. Benson and D. Blumer. New York: Grune & Stratton.

Bozeat, S., Lambon Ralph, M.A., Patterson, K., Garrard, P. and Hodges, J.R. (2000). Non-verbal semantic impairment in semantic dementia. *Neuropsychologia*, **38**, 1207–1215.

Brandt, J., Seidman, L.J. and Kohl, D. (1985). Personality characteristics of epileptic patients: a controlled study of generalized and temporal lobe cases. *Journal of Clinical and Experimental Neuropsychology*, **7**, 25–38.

Brekke, J.S., DeBonis, J.A. and Graham, J.W. (1994). A latent structure analysis of the positive and negative symptoms in schizophrenia. *Comprehensive Psychiatry*, **35**, 252–259.

Brekke, J.S., Raine, A. and Thomson, C. (1995). Cognitive and psychophysiological correlates of positive, negative, and disorganized symptoms in the schizophrenia spectrum. *Psychiatry Research*, **57**, 241–250.

Brown, G.W., Birley, J.L.T. and Wing, J.K. (1972). Influence of family life on the course of schizophrenic disorders: a replication. *British Journal of Psychiatry*, **121**, 241–258.

Brown, G.W., Carstairs, G.M. and Topping, G.C. (1958). The post hospital adjustment of chronic mental patients. *Lancet*, **ii**, 685–689.

Brown, G.W., Monck, E.M., Carstairs, G.M. and Wing, J.K. (1962). The influence of family life on the course of schizophrenic illness. *British Journal of Preventative and Social Medicine*, **16**, 55–68.

Brown, K.W. and White, T. (1992). Syndromes of chronic schizophrenia and some clinical correlates. *British Journal of Psychiatry*, **161**, 317–322.

Brüne, M. (2003). Theory of mind and the role of IQ in chronic disorganised schizophrenia. *Schizophrenia Research*, **60**, 57–64.

Buckingham, H.W., Jr. (1982). Can listeners draw implicatures from schizophrenics? *Behaviourial and Brain Sciences*, **5**, 592–594.

Burgess, P.W. and Shallice, T. (1997). *The Hayling and Brixton Tests*. Bury St Edmunds, Suffolk: Thames Valley Test Company.

Cadenhead, K.S., Geyer, M.A., Butler, R.W., Perry, W., Sprock, J. and Braff, D.L. (1997). Information processing deficits of schizophrenia patients: relationship to clinical ratings, gender and medication status. *Schizophrenia Research*, **28**, 51–62.

Cameron, N. (1938). Reasoning, regression and communication in schizophrenics. *Psychological Monographs*, **50**, 1–34.

(1939a). Deterioration and regression in schizophrenic thinking. *Journal of Abnormal and Social Psychology*, **34**, 265–270.

(1939b). Schizophrenic thinking in a problem-solving situation. *Journal of Mental Science*, **85**, 1012–1035.

Cameron, A.M., Oram, J., Geffen, G.M., Kavanagh, D.J., McGrath, J.J. and Geffen, L. (2002). Working memory correlates of three symptom clusters in schizophrenia. *Psychiatry Research*, **110**, 49–61.

Campbell, J.D. (1953). *Manic-Depressive Disease: Clinical and Psychiatric Significance.* Philadelphia: Lipincott.

Caraceni, A. and Grassi, L. (2003). *Delirium: Acute Confusional States in Palliative Medicine.* Oxford: Oxford University Press.

Cardno, A., Jones, L.A., Murphy, K.C., Asherson, P., Scott, L.C., Williams, J., Owen, M.J. and McGuffin, P. (1996). Factor analysis of schizophrenic symptoms using the OPCRIT checklist. *Schizophrenia Research*, **22**, 233–239.

Carlson, G.A. and Goodwin, F.K. (1973). The stages of mania: a longitudinal analysis of the manic episode. *Archives of General Psychiatry*, **28**, 221–228.

Carpenter, W.T., Bartko, J.J., Carpenter, C.L. and Strauss, J.L. (1976). Another view of schizophrenic subtypes. *Archives of General Psychiatry*, **33**, 508–516.

Chaika, E.O. (1974). A linguist looks at 'schizophrenic' language. *Brain and Language*, **1**, 257–276.

(1982). A unified explanation for the diverse structural deviations reported for adult schizophrenics with disrupted speech. *Journal of Communication Disorders*, **15**, 167–189.

(1990). *Understanding Psychotic Speech: Beyond Freud and Chomsky.* Springfield: Charles C. Thomas.

Chaika, E. and Alexander, P. (1986). The ice cream stories: a study in normal and psychotic narrations. *Discourse Processes*, **7**, 305–328.

Chaika, E.O. and Lambe, R.A. (1989). Cohesion in schizophrenic narratives, revisited. *Journal of Communication Disorders*, **22**, 407–421.

*Chapin, K., McCown, J., Vann, L., Kenney, D. and Youssef, I. (1992). Activation and facilitation in the lexicon of schizophrenics. *Schizophrenia Research*, **6**, 251–255.

Chapman, L.J. and Chapman, J.P. (1973). *Disordered Thought in Schizophrenia.* New York: Apple-Century-Crofts,.

Chapman, L.J., Chapman, J.P. and Miller, G.A. (1964). A theory of verbal behaviour in schizophrenia. In *Progress in Experimental Personality Research*, vol.1, ed. B.A. Maher. New York: Academic Press.

Chapman, L.J. and Taylor, J.A. (1957). Breadth of deviate concepts used by schizophrenics. *Journal of Abnormal and Social Psychology*, **54**, 118–123.

Chédru, F. and Geschwind, N. (1972). Disorders of higher cortical functions in acute confusional states. *Cortex*, **8**, 395–411.

Chua, S.E. and McKenna, P.J. (1995). Schizophrenia – a brain disease? A critical review of structural and functional cerebral abnormality in the disorder. *British Journal of Psychiatry*, **166**, 563–582.

Clare, L., McKenna, P.J., Mortimer, A.M. and Baddeley, A.D. (1993). Memory in schizophrenia: what is impaired and what is preserved? *Neuropsychologia*, **31**, 1225–1241.

Clark, H. and Haviland, S. (1977). Comprehension and the given-new contract. In *Discourse Production and Comprehension*, ed. R.O. Freedle. New Jersey: Ablex Publishing.

Clark, O. and O'Carroll, R.E. (1998). An examination of the relationship between executive function, memory and rehabilitation status in schizophrenia. *Neuropsychological Rehabilitation*, **8**, 229–241.

Clarke, P.R.F., Wyke, M. and Zangwill, O.L. (1958). Language disorder in a case of Korsakoff's syndrome. *Journal of Neurology, Neurosurgery and Psychiatry*, **21**, 190–194.

Cohen, B.D. (1978). Referent communication disturbances in schizophrenia. In *Language and Cognition in Schizophrenia*, ed. S. Schwartz. Hillsdale, New Jersey: Lawrence Erlbaum Associates.

Cohen, B.D. and Camhi, J. (1967). Schizophrenic performance in a word-communication task. *Journal of Abnormal Psychology*, **72**, 240–246.

Cohen, J.D. and Servan-Schreiber, D. (1992). Context, cortex and dopamine: a connectionist approach to behaviour and biology in schizophrenia. *Psychological Review*, **99** (1), 45–77.

Collins, A.M. and Loftus, E.F. (1975). A spreading-activation theory of semantic processing. *Psychological Review*, **82**, 407–428.

Collins, A.M. and Quillian, M.R. (1969). Retrieval time from semantic memory. *Journal of Verbal Learning and Verbal Memory*, **8**, 240–247.

*Condray, R., Steinhauer, S.R., Cohen, J.D., van Kammen, D.P. and Kasparek, A. (1999). Modulation of language processing in schizophrenia: effects of context and haloperidol on the event-related potential. *Biological Psychiatry*, **45**, 1336–1355.

Conti-Ramsden, G., Crutchley, A. and Botting, N. (1997). The extent to which psychometric tests differentiate subgroups of children with SLI. *Journal of Speech, Language and Hearing Research*, **40**, 765–777.

Cooper, J.E., Kendell, R.E., Gurland, B.J., Sharpe, L., Copeland, J.R.M. and Simon, R. (1972). *Psychiatric Diagnosis in New York and London: A Comparative Study of Mental Hospital Admissions* (Maudsley Monograph, 20). London: Oxford University Press.

Corcoran, R. and Frith, C.D.(1996). Conversational conduct and the symptoms of schizophrenia. *Cognitive Neuropsychiatry*, **1**, 305–318.

Corcoran, R., Cahill, C. and Frith, C.D. (1997). The appreciation of visual jokes in people with schizophrenia: a study of 'mentalizing' ability. *Schizophrenia Research*, **24**, 319–327.

Corcoran, R., Mercer, G. and Frith, C.D. (1995). Schizophrenia, symptomatology and social inference: Investigating 'theory of mind' in people with schizophrenia. *Schizophrenia Research*, **17**, 5–13.

Crawford, J.R., Obonswain, M.C. and Bremner, M. (1993). Frontal lobe impairment in schizophrenia: relationship to intellectual functioning. *Psychological Medicine*, **23**, 787–790.

Critchley, M. (1964). The neurology of psychotic speech. *British Journal of Psychiatry*, **110**, 353–364.

Crow, T.J. (1980). Molecular pathology of schizophrenia: more than one disease process? *British Medical Journal*, **280**, 66–68.

Crow, T.J. and Mitchell, W.S. (1975). Subjective age in chronic schizophrenia: evidence for a subgroup of patients with defective learning capacity. *British Journal of Psychiatry*, **126**, 360–363.

Cuesta, M.J. and Peralta, V. (1995). Cognitive disorders in the positive, negative and disorganization syndromes of schizophrenia. *Psychiatry Research*, **58**, 227–235.

Curran, F.J. and Schilder, P. (1935). Paraphasic signs in diffuse lesions of the brain. *Journal of Nervous and Mental Disease*, **82**, 613–636.

Cutting, J. (1980). Physical illness and psychosis. *British Journal of Psychiatry*, **136**, 109–119.

(1985). *The Psychology of Schizophrenia*. Edinburgh: Churchill Livingstone.

(1987). The phenomenology of acute organic psychoses: comparison with acute schizophrenia. *British Journal of Psychiatry*, **151**, 324–332.

Daban, C., Amado, I., Baylé, F., Gut, A., Willard, D., Bourdel, M.-C., Loo, H., Olié, J.-P., Millet, B., Krebs, M.-O. and Poirier, M.-F. (2002). Correlation between clinical syndromes and neurological tasks in unmedicated patients with recent onset schizophrenia. *Psychiatry Research*, **113**, 83–92.

David, A.S. (1992). Frontal lobology – psychiatry's new pseudoscience. *British Journal of Psychiatry*, **161**, 244–248.

Davidson, L.L. and Heinrichs, R.W. (2003). Quantification of frontal and temporal lobe brain-imaging findings in schizophrenia: a meta-analysis. *Psychiatry Research: Neuroimaging*, **122**, 69–87.

De Renzi, E. and Faglioni, P. (1978). Normative data and screening power of a shortened version of the token test. *Cortex*, **14**, 41–49.

de Vries, P.J., Honer, W.G., Kemp, P.M. and McKenna, P.J. (2001). Dementia as a complication of schizophrenia. *Journal of Neurology, Neurosurgery and Psychiatry*, **70**, 588–596.

Diem, O. (1903). Die einfach demente Form der Dementia Praecox. Dementia simplex. *Archiv für psychiatrie and Nervenkrankheiten*, **37**, 111–187. [Partly translated (1987) as 'Simple schizophrenia'. In *The Clinical Roots of the Schizophrenia Concept*, ed. J. Cutting and M. Shepherd. Cambridge: Cambridge University Press.]

Docherty, N.M., Cohen, A.S., Nienow, T.M., Dinzeo, T.J. and Dangelmaier, R.E. (2003). Stability of formal thought disorder and referential communication disturbances in schizophrenia. *Journal of Abnormal Psychology*, **112**(3), 469–475.

Docherty, N.M. and Gordinier, S.W. (1999). Immediate memory, attention and communication disturbances in schizophrenia patients and their relatives. *Psychological Medicine*, **29**, 189–197.

Docherty, N.M. and Gottesman, I. (2000). A twin study of communication disturbances in schizophrenia. *Journal of Nervous and Mental Disorders*, **188**, 395–401.

Docherty, N.M., Hawkins, K.A., Hoffman, R.E., Quinlan, D.M., Rakfeldt, J. and Sledge, W.H. (1996). Working memory, attention, and communication disturbances in schizophrenia. *Journal of Abnormal Psychology*, **105**, 212–219.

Docherty, N.M., Schnur, M. and Harvey, P.D. (1988). Reference performance and positive and negative thought disorder: a follow-up study of manics and schizophrenics. *Journal of Abnormal Psychology*, **97**, 437–442.

Dollfus, S. and Everitt, B. (1998). Symptom structure in schizophrenia: two-, three- or four-factor models. *Psychopathology*, **31**, 120–130.

Doody, G.A., Gotz, M., Johnstone, E.C., Frith, C.D. and Owens, D.G. (1998). Theory of mind and psychoses. *Psychological Medicine*, **28**, 397–405.

Drury, V.M., Robinson, E.J. and Birchwood, M. (1998) 'Theory of mind' skills during an acute episode of psychosis and following recovery. *Psychological Medicine*, **28**, 1101–1112.

Durbin, M. and Martin, R.L. (1977). Speech in mania: syntactic aspects. *Brain and Language*, **4**, 208–218.

Eckman, P.S. and Shean, G.D. (2000). Impairment in test performance and symptom dimensions of schizophrenia. *Journal of Psychiatric Research*, **34**, 147–153.

Elliott, R., McKenna, P.J., Robbins, T.W. and Sahakian, B.J. (1995). Neuropsychological evidence of frontostriatal dysfunction in schizophrenia. *Psychological Medicine*, **25**, 619–630. (1998). Specific neuropsychologcial deficits in schizophrenic patients with perserved intellectual function. *Cognitive Neuropsychiatry*, **3**, 45–70.

Ellman, R. (1959). *James Joyce*. New York: Oxford University Press.

Epstein, S. (1953). Overinclusive thinking in a schizophrenic and a control group. *Journal of Consulting Psychology*, **17**, 384–388.

Evans, J., Chua, S., McKenna, P. and Wilson, B. (1997). Assessment of the dysexecutive syndrome in schizophrenia. *Psychological Medicine*, **27**, 635–646.

Faber, R., Abrams, R., Taylor, M.A., Kasprison, A., Morris, C. and Weisz, R. (1983). Comparison of schizophrenic patients with formal thought disorder and neurologically impaired patients with aphasia. *American Journal of Psychiatry*, **140**, 1348–1351.

Faber, R. and Reichstein, M.B. (1981). Language dysfunction in schizophrenia. *British Journal of Psychiatry*, **139**, 519–522.

Fish, F.J. (1957). The classification of schizophrenia: the views of Kleist and his co-workers. *Journal of Mental Science*, **103**, 443–463.

Fitzgerald, M. (2004). *Autism and Creativity*. Hove: Brunner-Routledge.

Folstein, M.F., Folstein, S.E. and McHugh, P.R. (1975). 'Mini-Mental State': a practical method for grading the cognitive state of patients for the clinician. *Journal of Psychiatric Research*, **12**, 189–198

Forrest, D.V. (1965). Poiesis and the language of schizophrenia. *Psychiatry*, **28**, 1–18.

Fraser, W.I., King, K.M., Thomas, P. and Kendell, R.E. (1986). The diagnosis of schizophrenia by language analysis. *British Journal of Psychiatry*, **148**, 275–278.

Frith, C.D. (1987). The positive and negative symptoms of schizophrenia reflect impairments in the perception and initiation of action. *Psychological Medicine*, **17**, 631–648. (1992). *The Cognitive Neuropsychology of Schizophrenia*. Hove: Lawrence Erlbaum Associates. (1999). Commentary on laws: what are we trying to explain? *Cognitive Neuropsychiatry*, **4**, 31–32.

Frith, C.D and Corcoran, R. (1996). Exploring 'theory of mind' in people with schizophrenia. *Psychological Medicine*, **26**, 521–530.

Frith, C.D., Leary, J., Cahill, C. and Johnstone, E.C. (1991). Performance on psychological tests. Demographic and clinical correlates of the results of these tests. *British Journal of Psychiatry*, **159**, Supplement, **13**, 26–29.

Frith, U. (2003). *Autism: Explaining the Enigma*, 2nd edn. Oxford: Blackwell.

Fromkin, V.A. (1975). 'A linguist looks at schizophrenic language'. *Brain and Language*, **2**, 498–503.

Garrard, P. and Hodges, J.R. (1999). Semantic dementia: implications for the neural basis of language and meaning. *Aphasiology*, **13**, 609–623.

Gastaut, H. (1954). Interpretation of the symptoms of psychomotor epilepsy in relation to physiological data on rhinencephalic function. *Epilepsia*, **3**, 84–88.

Gastaut, H. and Collomb, H. (1954). Etude de comportemente sexual chez les épileptiques psychomoteurs. *Annales Médico-Psychologique*, **112**, 657–696.

Gastaut, H., Roger, J. and Lesevre, N. (1953). Différenciation psychologique des épileptiques en fonction des formes électrocliniques de leur maladie. *Revue de Psychologie Appliquée*, **3**, 237–249.

Geschwind, N. (1979). Behavioural changes in temporal lobe epilepsy. *Psychological Medicine*, **9**, 217–219.

Glucksberg, S., Krauss, R.M. and Higgins, E. (1975). The development of referential communication skills. *Review of Child Development Research*, ed. F. Horowitz, Vol. IV, pp. 305–346. Chicago: Chicago University Press.

Goldberg, T.E., and Gold, J.M. (1995). Neurocognitive deficits in schizophrenia. In *Schizophrenia*, ed. S.R. Hirsch and D.R. Weinberger. Oxford: Blackwell.

Goldberg, T.E., Aloia, M.S., Gourevitch, M.L., Missar, D., Pickar, D. and Weinberger, D.R. (1998). Cognitive substrates of thought disorder: I. The semantic system. *American Journal of Psychiatry*, **155**, 1671–1676.

Goldberg, T.E., Kelsoe, J.R., Weinberger, D.R., Pliskin, N.H., Kirwin, P.D. and Berman, K.F. (1988). Performance of schizophrenic patients on putative neuropsychological tests of frontal lobe function. *International Journal of Neuroscience*, **42**, 51–58.

Goldberg, T.E. and Weinberger, D.R. (2000). Thought disorder in schizophrenia: a reappraisal of older formulations and an overview of some recent studies. *Cognitive Neuropsychiatry*, **5**, 1–19.

Goldberg, T.E., Weinberger, D.R., Berman, K.F., Pliskin, N.H. and Podd, M.H. (1987). Further evidence for dementia of prefrontal type in schizophrenia? A controlled study of teaching the Wisconsin Card Sorting Test. *Archives of General Psychiatry*, **44**, 1008–1014.

Goldstein, K. (1944). Methodological approach to the study of schizophrenic thought disorder. In *Language and Thought in Schizophrenia*, ed. J.S. Kasanin. Berkeley/Los Angeles: University of California Press.

Goodglass, H. and Kaplan, E. (1994). *The Assessment of Aphasia and Related Disorders*, 2nd edn. Philadelphia: Lea & Febiger.

Goodwin, F.K. and Jamison, K.R. (1990). *Manic-Depressive Illness*. New York: Oxford University Press.

*Gouzoulis-Mayfrank, E., Voss, T., Mörth, T., Thelen, B., Spitzer, M. and Meincke, U. (2003). Semantic hyperpriming in thought-disordered patients with schizophrenia: state or trait? – a longitudinal investigation. *Schizophrenia Research*, **65**, 65–73.

Graham, K.S. and Hodges, J.R. (1997). Differentiating the roles of the hippocampal system and the neocortex in long-term memory storage. *Neuropsychology*, **11**, 77–89.

Gray, J.A. and McNaughton, N. (2000). *The Neuropsychology of Anxiety: An Enquiry into the Functions of the Septo-Hippocampal System*, 2nd edn. Oxford: Oxford University Press.

Grice, H.P. (1957). Meaning. *The Philosophical Review*, **62**, 377–388.

(1975). Logic and conversation. In *Syntax and Semantics*, ed. P. Cole and J.P. Morgan. New York: Seminar Press.

Guillem, F., Bicu, M., Bloom, D., Wolf, M.-A., Desautels, R., Lalinec, M., Krause, D. and Debruille, J.B. (2001). Neuropsychological impairments in the syndromes of schizophrenia: a comparison between different dimensional models. *Brain and Cognition*, **46**, 153–159.

Gureje, O., Aderibigbe, Y.A. and Obikaya, O. (1995). Three syndromes in schizophrenia: validity in young patients with a recent onset of illness. *Psychological Medicine*, **25**, 715–725.

Gustafson, L. (1987). Frontal lobe degeneration of non-Alzheimer type. II. Clinical picture and differential diagnosis. *Archives of Gerontology and Geriatrics*, **6**, 209–223.

Halliday, M.A.K. and Hasan, R. (1976). *Cohesion in English*. London: Longman.

Harrow, M. and Miller, J.G. (1980). Schizophrenic thought disorders and impaired perspective. *Journal of Abnormal Psychology*, **89**, 717–727.

Harrow, M. and Prosen, M. (1978). Intermingling and disordered logic as influences on schizophrenic 'thought disorders'. *Archives of General Psychiatry*, **35**, 1213–1218.

(1979). Schizophrenic thought disorders: bizarre associations and intermingling. *American Journal of Psychiatry*, **136**, 293–296.

Harrow, M. and Quinlan, D. (1977). Is disordered thinking unique to schizophrenia? *Archives of General Psychiatry*, **34**, 15–21.

(1985). *Disordered Thinking and Schizophrenic Psychopathology*. New York: Gardner Press.

Harrow, M., Adler, D. and Hanf, E. (1974). Abstract and concrete thinking in schizophrenia during the prechronic phases. *Archives of General Psychiatry*, **31**, 27–33.

Harrow, M., Harkavy, K., Bromet, E. and Tucker, G.J. (1973). A longitudinal study of schizophrenic thinking. *Archives of General Psychiatry*, **28**, 179–182.

Harrow, M., Tucker, G.J. and Shield, P. (1972a). Stimulus overinclusion in schizophrenic disorders. *Archives of General Psychiatry*, **27**, 40–45.

Harrow, M., Himmelhoch, J.M., Tucker, G.J., Hersh, J. and Quinlan, D. (1972b). Overinclusive thinking in acute schizophrenic patients. *Journal of Abnormal Psychology*, **79**, 161–168.

Harrow, M., Lanin-Kettering, I., Prosen, M. and Miller, J.G. (1983). Disordered thinking in schizophrenia: intermingling and loss of set. *Schizophrenia Bulletin*, **9**, 354–367.

Harrow, M., Quinlan, D., Wallington, S. and Pickett, L.Jr. (1976). Primitive drive-dominated thinking: relationship to acute schizophrenia and sociopathy. *Journal of Personality Assessment*, **40**, 31–41.

Harvey, P.D. (1983). Speech competence in manic and schizophrenic psychoses: the association between clinically related thought disorder and cohesion and reference performance. *Journal of Abnormal Psychology*, **92**, 368–377.

Harvey, P.D., Earle-Boyer, E.A. and Wielgus, M.S. (1984). The consistency of thought disorder in mania and schizophrenia. *Journal of Nervous and Mental Disease*, **172**, 458–463.

Harvey, P.D., Lenzenwegger, M.F., Keefe, R.S.E., Pogge, D.L., Serper, M.R. and Mohs, R.C. (1992). Empirical assessment of the factorial structure of clinical symptoms in schizophrenic patients: formal thought disorder. *Psychiatry Research*, **44**, 141–151.

Hawks, D.V. and Payne, R.W. (1971). Overinclusive thought disorder and symptomatology. *British Journal of Psychiatry*, **118**, 663–670.

Heaton, R. K, Baade, L. E. and Johnson, K.L. (1978). Neuropsychological test results associated with psychiatric disorders in adults. *Psychological Bulletin*, **85**, 141–162.

Heinrichs, R.W. (2001). *In Search of Madness*. New York: Oxford University Press.

Heinrichs, R.W. and Zakzanis, K.K. (1998). Neurocognitive deficit in schizophrenia: a quantitative review of the evidence. *Neuropsychology*, **12**, 426–445.

*Henik, A., Nissimov, E., Priel, B. and Umansky, R. (1995). Effects of cognitive load on semantic priming in patients with schizophrenia. *Journal of Abnormal Psychology*, **104**, 576–584.

*Henik, A., Priel, B. and Umansky, R. (1992). Attention and automaticity in semantic processing of schizophrenic patients. *Neuropsychiatry, Neuropsychology, and Behavioral Neurology*, **5**, 161–169.

Herbert, R.K. and Waltensperger, K.Z. (1980). Schizophrasia: case study of a paranoid schizophrenic's language. *Applied Psycholinguistics*, **1**, 81–93.

Hermann, B.P. and Riel, P. (1981). Interictal personality and behavioral traits in temporal lobe and generalized epilepsy. *Cortex*, **17**, 125–128.

Hill, K.E., Mann, L., Laws. K.R., Stevenson, C.M.E., Nimmo-Smith, I. and McKenna, P.J. (2004). Hypofrontality in schizophrenia: a meta-analysis of functional imaging studies. *Acta Psychiatrica Scandinavica*, **110**, 243–256.

Himelhoch, S., Taylor, S.F., Goldman, R.S. and Tandon, R. (1996). Frontal lobe tasks, antipsychotic medication and schizophrenia syndromes. *Biological Psychiatry*, **39**, 227–229.

Hodges, J.R. (1993). Pick's disease: its relationship to semantic dementia, progressive aphasia and frontotemporal dementia. In *Dementia*, ed. A. Burns and R. Levy. London: Chapman & Hall.

Hodges, J.R. and Patterson, K. (1997). Semantic memory disorders. *Trends in Cognitive Sciences*, **1**, 68–72.

Hodges, J.R., Patterson, K., Oxbury, S. and Funnell, E. (1992). Semantic dementia: progressive fluent aphasia with temporal lobe atrophy. *Brain*, **115**, 1783–1806.

Hoff, E. (2001). *Language Development*. California: Wadsworth.

Hoffman, R. and Sledge, W. (1984). A microgenetic model of paragrammatisms produced by a schizophrenic speaker. *Brain and Language*, **21**, 147–173.

Hoffman, R.E. and Sledge, W. (1988). An analysis of grammatical deviance occurring in spontaneous schizophrenic speech. *Journal of Neurolinguistics*, **3**, 89–101.

Howard, D. and Patterson, K.E. (1992). *The Pyramids and Palm Trees Test: A Test of Semantic Access from Pictures and Words*. Bury St Edmunds: Thames Valley Test Co.

Humphreys, G.W. and Riddoch, M.J. (1987). *To See but Not to See: A Case Study of Visual Agnosia*. Hove: Erlbaum.

Hunt, M. (1997). *How Science Takes Stock*. New York: Russell Sage Foundation.

Ianzito, B.M., Cadoret, R.J. and Pugh, D.D. (1974). Thought disorder in depression. *American Journal of Psychiatry*, **131**, 703–707.

Ingvar, D.H. and Franzen, G. (1974). Abnormalities of cerebral blood flow distribution in patients with chronic schizophrenia. *Acta Psychiatrica Scandinavica*, **50**, 425–462.

James, I. (2003). Singular scientists. *Journal of the Royal Society of Medicine*, **96**, 36–39.

Jamison, K.R. (1993). *Touched with Fire: Manic Depressive Illness and the Artistic Temperament*. New York: Free Press.

Johnstone, E.C. and Frith, C.D. (1996). Validation of three dimensions of schizophrenic symptoms in a large unselected sample of patients. *Psychological Medicine*, 26, 669–679.

Johnstone, E.C., Crow, T.J., Frith, C.D., Carney, M.W.P. and Price, J.S. (1978). Mechanism of the antipsychotic effect in the treatment of acute schizophrenia. *Lancet*, i, 848–851.

Johnstone, E.C., Crow, T.J., Frith, C.D., Husband, J. and Kreel, L. (1976). Cerebral ventricular size and cognitive impairment in chronic schizophrenia. *Lancet*, ii, 924–926.

Joyce, E., Collinson, S.L. and Crichton, P. (1996). Verbal fluency in schizophrenia: relationship with executive function, semantic memory and clinical alogia. *Psychological Medicine*, 26, 39–49.

Kaczmarek, B.L.J. (1984). Neurolinguistic analysis of verbal utterances in patients with focal lesions of the frontal lobes. *Brain and Language*, 21, 52–58.

Kahlbaum, K.L. (1874). *Catatonia* (trans. Y. Levij and T. Priden, 1973). Baltimore: Johns Hopkins University Press.

Kay, S.R. and Sevy, S. (1990). Pyramidical model of schizophrenia. *Schizophrenia Bulletin*, 16, 537–545.

Kendell, R.E. (1975). *The Role of Diagnosis in Psychiatry*. Oxford: Blackwell.

King, D.J. (1990). The effect of neuroleptics on cognitive and psychomotor function. *British Journal of Psychiatry*, 157, 799–811.

Kintsch, W. (1980). Semantic memory: a tutorial. In *Attention and Performance*, VIII, ed. R.S. Nickerson. Hillsdale, NJ: Erlbaum.

Kitselman, K. (1981). Language impairment in aphasia, delirium, dementia, and schizophrenia. In *Speech Evaluation in Medicine*, ed. J.K. Darby. New York: Grune & Stratton.

Kleist, K. (1914). Aphasia and Geisteskrankheit. *Münchener Medizinische Wochenschrift*, 61, 8–12. (1930). Zur hirnpathologischen Auffassung der schizophrenen Grundstörungen. Die alogische Denkstörung. *Schweizer Archiv für Neurologie und Psychiatrie*, 26, 99–102. [Translated (1987) as: Alogical thought disorder: an organic manifestation of the schizophrenic psychological deficit. In *The Clinical Roots of the Schizophrenia Concept*, ed. J. Cutting and M. Shepherd. Cambridge: Cambridge University Press.] (1960). Schizophrenic symptoms and cerebral pathology. *Journal of Mental Science*, 106, 246–255.

Kraepelin, E. (1896). Dementia praecox. In *The Clinical Roots of the Schizophrenia Concept*, ed. J. Cutting and M. Shepherd (1987). Cambridge: Cambridge University Press. (1907). *Clinical Psychiatry*, 7th edn (trans. A.R. Diefendorf, 1915). New York: Macmillan. (1913a). *Dementia Praecox and Paraphrenia* (trans. R.M. Barclay, 1919). Edinburgh: Livingstone. (1913b). *Manic-Depressive Insanity and Paranoia* (trans. R.M. Barclay, 1921). Edinburgh: Livingstone. (1923). *Psychiatrie*, ed. 8. Leipzig: Barth.

Küfferle, B., Lenz, G. and Schanda, H. (1985). Clinical evaluation of language and thought disorders in patients with schizophrenic and affective psychoses. *Psychopathology*, 18, 126–132.

Kuperberg, G.R., McGuire, P.K. and David, A. (1998). Reduced sensitivity to linguistic context in schizophrenic thought disorder: evidence from on-line monitoring for words in linguistically anomalous sentences. *Journal of Abnormal Psychology*, 107, 423–434.

Landre, N.A., Taylor, M.A. and Kearns, K.P. (1992). Language functioning in schizophrenic and aphasic patients. *Neuropsychiatry, Neuropsychology and Behavioral Neurology*, **5**, 7–14.

Langdon, R., Coltheart, M., Ward, P.B. and Catts, S.V. (2002) Disturbed communication in schizophrenia: the role of poor pragmatics and poor mind-reading. *Psychological Medicine*, **32**, 1273–1284.

Laws, K.R. (1999). A meta-analytic review of Wisconsin Card Sort studies in schizophrenia: general intellectual deficit in disguise? *Cognitive Neuropsychiatry*, **4**, 1–30.

Laws, K.R., Al-Uzri, M. and Mortimer, A.M. (2000). Lexical knowledge degradation in schizophrenia. *Schizophrenia Research*, **45**, 123–131.

Laws, K.R., Humber, S.A., Ramsey, D.J.C. and McCarthy, R.A. (1995a). Probing sensory and associative semantics for animals and objects in normal subjects. *Memory*, **3**, 397–408.

Laws, K.R., Evans, J.J., Hodges J.R. and McCarthy, R.M. (1995b). Naming without knowing and appearance without associations: evidence for constructive processes in semantic memory? *Memory*, **3**, 409–433.

Laws, K.R. Kondel, T.K. and McKenna, P.J. (1999). A receptive language deficit in schizophrenic thought disorder: evidence for impaired semantic access and monitoring. *Cognitive Neuropsychiatry*, **4**, 89–105.

Laws, K. Mckenna, P.J. and Kondel, T. (1998). On the distinction between access and store disorders in schizophrenia: a question of deficit severity? *Neuropsychologia*, **36**, 313–321.

Lecours, A.R. and Vanier-Clément, M. (1976). Schizophasia and jargonaphasia: a comparative description with comments on Chaika's and Fromkin's respective looks at 'schizophrenic' language. *Brain and Language*, **3**, 516–565.

Leonhard, K. (1979). *The Classification of Endogenous Psychoses*, 5th edn (trans. R. Berman). New York: Irvington.

Levinson, S.C. (1983). *Pragmatics*. Cambridge: Cambridge University Press.

Lewis, A.J. (1934). Melancholia: a clinical survey of depressive states. *Journal of Mental Science*, **80**, 277–378. [Reprinted 1967, in *Inquiries in Psychiatry: Clinical and Social Investigations*. London: Routledge & Kegan Paul.]

Lidderdale, J. (1983). Lucia Joyce at St Andrew's. *James Joyce Broadsheet*, Number 11.

Liddle, P.F. (1987a). The symptoms of chronic schizophrenia: a re-examination of the positive-negative dichotomy. *British Journal of Psychiatry*, **151**, 145–151.

(1987b). Schizophrenic syndromes, cognitive performance and neurological dysfunction. *Psychological Medicine*, **17**, 49–57.

(1995). *Thought Language and Communication Index*. Vancouver: Department of Psychiatry, Universities of Vancouver.

Liddle, P.F. and Barnes, T.R.E. (1990). Syndromes of chronic schizophrenia. *British Journal of Psychiatry*, **157**, 558–561.

Liddle, P.F. and Crow, T.J. (1984). Age disorientation in chronic schizophrenia is associated with global intellectual impairment. *British Journal of Psychiatry*, **144**, 193–199.

Liddle, P.F. and Morris, D.L. (1991). Schizophrenic syndromes and frontal lobe performance. *British Journal of Psychiatry*, **158**, 340–345.

Lipowski, Z.J. (1990). *Delirium: Acute Confusional States*. New York/Oxford: Oxford University Press.

Lishman. W.A. (1998). *Organic Psychiatry*, 3rd edn. Oxford: Blackwell Science.

Lorenz, M. (1968). Problems posed by schizophrenic language. In *Language Behavior in Schizophrenia*, ed. H.J. Vetter. Springfield, Illinois: Charles C. Thomas.

Maher, B.A. (1983). A tentative theory of schizophrenic utterance. In *Progress in Experimental Personality Research, vol. 12: Personality*, ed. B.A. Maher and W.B. Maher. New York: Academic Press.

Malla, A.K., Ross, M.G., Norman, P.W., Cortese, L. and Diaz, F. (1993). Three syndrome concept of schizophrenia: a factor analytic study. *Schizophrenia Research*, 10, 143–150.

Malmkjaer, K. (1991). *The Linguistics Encyclopedia*. London: Routledge.

Manschreck, T.C., Maher, B.A., Milavetz, J.J., Ames, D., Weinstein, C.C. and Schneyer, M.L. (1988). Semantic priming in thought disordered schizophrenic patients. *Schizophrenia Research*, 1, 61–66.

Master, D.R., Toone, B.K. and Scott, D.F. (1984). Interictal behaviour in temporal lobe epilepsy. In *Advances in Epileptology: The XVth Epilepsy International Symposium*, ed. R. J. Porter, R.H. Mattson, A.A. Ward, Jr. and M. Dam. New York: Raven Press.

Mazza, M., De Risio, A., Surian, L., Roncone, R. and Casacchia, M. (2001). Selective impairments of theory of mind in people with schizophrenia. *Schizophrenia Research*, 47, 299–308.

McGrath, J. (1991). Ordering thoughts on thought disorder. *British Journal of Psychiatry*, 158, 307–316.

McKay, A.P., McKenna, P.J., Mortimer, A.M., Bentham, P. and Hodges, J.R. (1996). Semantic memory is impaired in schizophrenia. *Biological Psychiatry*, 39, 929–937.

McKenna, P.J. (1994). *Schizophrenia and Related Syndromes*. Oxford: Oxford University Press.

McKenna, P.J. and Laws, K. (1997). Schizophrenic amnesia. In *Case Studies in the Neuropsychology of Memory*, ed. A. Parkin. Hove: Psychology Press.

McKenna, P.J. Ornstein, T. and Baddeley, A.D. (2002). Schizophrenia. In *Handbook of Memory Disorders*, 2nd edn, ed. A. D Baddeley, B.A. Wilson and M. Kopelman. Chichester: Wiley.

Mey, J.L. (2001) *Pragmatics: An Introduction*, 2nd edn. Oxford: Blackwell.

Miller, B. (1974). Semantic misinterpretation of ambiguous communications in schizophrenia. *Archives of General Psychiatry*, 30, 435–440.

Miller, D.D., Arndt, S. and Andreasen, N.C. (1993). Alogia, attentional impairment, and inappropriate affect: their status in the dimensions of schizophrenia. *Comprehensive Psychiatry*, 34, 221–226.

Minzenberg, M., Ober, B.A. and Vinogradov, S. (2002). Semantic priming in schizophrenia: a review and synthesis. *Journal of the International Neuropsychological Society*, 8, 699–720.

Minzenberg, M.J., Poole, J.H., Vinogradov, S., Shenaut, G.K. and Ober, B.A. (2003). Slowed lexical access is uniquely associated with positive and disorganised symptoms in schizophrenia. *Cognitive Neuropsychiatry*, 8, 107–128.

Mohamed, S., Paulsen, J.S., O'Leary, D., Arndt, S. and Andreasen, N.C. (1999). Generalized cognitive deficits in schizophrenia: a study of first episode patients. *Archives of General Psychiatry*, **56**, 749–754.

Moran, L.J. (1953). Vocabulary knowledge and usage among normal and schizophrenic subjects. *Psychological Monographs*, **67**, 1–19.

Morice, R. and Ingram, J.C.L. (1982). Language analysis in schizophrenia: diagnostic implications. *Australian and New Zealand Journal of Psychiatry*, **16**, 11–21.

Morice, R. and McNicol, D. (1985). The comprehension and production of complex syntax in schizophrenia. *Cortex*, **21**, 567–580.

Moritz, S., Andresen, B., Jacobsen, D., Mersmann, K., Wilke, U., Lambert, M., Naber, D. and Krausz, M. (2001). Neuropsychological correlates of schizophrenic syndromes in patients treated with atypical neuroleptics. *European Psychiatry*, **16**, 354–361.

*Moritz, S., Mersmann, K., Kloss, M., Jacobsen, D., Wilke, U., Andresen, B., Naber, D. and Pawlik, K. (2001). Hyper-priming in thought-disordered schizophrenic patients. *Psychological Medicine*, **31**, 221–229.

*Moritz, S., Woodward, T.S., Küppers, D., Lausen, A. and Schickel, M. (2002). Increased automatic spreading activation in thought-disordered schizophrenic patients. *Schizophrenia Research*, **59**, 181–186.

Mortimer, A.M. (1997). Cognitive function in schizophrenia: do neuroleptics make a difference. *Pharmacology, Biochemistry and Behavior*, **56**, 789–795.

Moscovitch, M. (1989). Confabulation and the frontal systems: strategic versus associative retrieval in neuropsychological theories of memory. In *Varieties of Memory and Consciousness*, ed. H.L. Roediger III and F.I. M Craik. Hillsdale, NJ: Erlbaum.

(1995). Confabulation. In *Memory Distortion*, ed. D.L. Schacter. Cambridge, MA: Harvard University Press.

Moscovitch, M. and Melo, B. (1997). Strategic retrieval and the frontal lobes: evidence from confabulation and amnesia. *Neuropsychologia*, **35**, 1017–1034.

Mourer, S. (1971). Some issues regarding semantic generalization in schizophrenics. *Proceedings of the Annual Convention of the American Psychological Association*, **6**, 449–450.

Mungas, D. (1982). Interictal behavioral abnormality in temporal lobe epilepsy: a specific syndrome or nonspecific psychopathology. *Archives of General Psychiatry*, **39**, 108–111.

Neary, D., Snowden, J.S., Northen, B. and Goulding, P. (1988). Dementia of frontal lobe type. *Journal of Neurology, Neurosurgery and Psychiatry*, **51**, 353–361.

Nelson, H.E. (1982). *The National Adult Reading Test (NART)*. Windsor: NFER-Nelson.

Nettle, D. (2001). *Stong Imagination: Madness, Creativity, and Human Nature*. Oxford: Oxford University Press.

Neuringer, C., Goldstein, G. and Fiske, J.P. (1969). Schizophrenic adherence to strong meaning associations. *Perceptual and Motor Skills*, **29**, 394.

Norman, D.A. and Shallice, T. (1980). *Attention to Action: Willed and Automatic Control of Behavior*. San Diego: University of California at San Diego, CHIP Report 99.

Norman, R.M.G., Malla, A.K., Morrison-Stewart, S.L., Helmes, E., Williamson, P.C., Thomas, J. and Cortese, L. (1997). Neuropsychological correlates of syndromes in schizophrenia. *British Journal of Psychiatry*, **170**, 134–139.

Novoa, O.P. and Ardila, A. (1987). Linguistic abilities in patients with prefrontal damage. *Brain and Language*, **30**, 206–225.

O'Leary, D.S., Flaum, M., Kesler, M.L., Flashman, L.A., Arndt, S. and Andreasen N.C. (2000). Cognitive correlates of negative, disorganized and psychotic symptom dimensions of schizophrenia. *Journal of Neuropsychiatry and Clinical Neurosciences*, **12**, 4–15.

*Ober, B.A., Vinogradov, S. and Shenaut, G.K. (1995). Semantic priming of category relations in schizophrenia. *Neuropsychology*, **9**, 220–228.

*Ober, B.A., Vinogradov, S. and Shenaut, G.K. (1997). Automatic versus controlled semantic priming in schizophrenia. *Neuropsychology*, **11**, 506–513.

Oh, T.M., McCarthy, R.A. and McKenna, P.J. (2002). Is there a schizophasia? A study applying the single case study approach to formal thought disorder in schizophrenia. *Neurocase*, **8**, 233–244.

Oltmanns, T.F., Murphy, R., Berenbaum, H. and Dunlop, S.A. (1985). Rating verbal communication impairment in schizophrenia and affective disorders. *Schizophrenia Bulletin*, **11**, 292–299.

Owens, D.G.C. and Johnstone, E.C. (1980). The disabilities of chronic schizophrenia – their nature and the factors contributing to their development. *British Journal of Psychiatry*, **136**, 384–393.

*Passerieux, C., Segui, J., Besche, C., Chevalier, J.F., Widlocher, D. and Hardy-Bayle, M.C. (1997). Heterogeneity in cognitive functioning of schizophrenic patients evaluated by a lexical decision task. *Psychological Medicine*, **27**, 1295–1302.

Payne, R.W. (1960). Cognitive abnormalities. In *Handbook of Abnormal Psychology*, ed. H.J. Eysenck. London: Pitman.

(1973). Cognitive abnormalities. In *Handbook of Abnormal Psychology*, 2nd edn, ed. H.J. Eysenck. London: Pitman.

Peralta, V., Cuesta, M.J. and de Leon, J. (1992). Formal thought disorder in schizophrenia: a factor analytic study. *Comprehensive Psychiatry*, **33**, 105–110.

(1994). An empirical analysis of latent structures underlying schizophrenic symptoms: a four-syndrome model. *Biological Psychiatry*, **36**, 726–736.

Perry, W., Heaton, R.K., Potterat, E., Roebuck, T., Minassian, A. and Braff, D.L. (2001). Working memory in schizophrenia: transient 'online' storage versus executive functioning. *Schizophrenia Bulletin*, **27**, 157–176.

Petrie, A. (1952). *Personality and the Frontal Lobes: An Investigation of the Psychological Effects of Different Types of Leucotomy*. London: Routledge & Kegan Paul.

Phillips, M.R., Xiong, W., Wang, R.W., Gao, Y.H., Wang, X.Q. and Zhang, N.P. (1991). Reliability and validity of the Chinese versions of the scales for the assessment of positive and negative symptoms. *Acta Psychiatrica Scandinavica*, **84**, 364–370.

Pickup, G.J. and Frith, C.D. (2001). Theory of mind impairments in schizophrenia: symptomatology, severity and specificity. *Psychological Medicine*, **31**, 207–220.

Pollice, R., Roncone, R., Falloon, I.R.H., Mazza, M., De Risio, A., Necozione, S., Morosini, P. and Casacchia, M. (2002). Is theory of mind in schizophrenia more strongly associated with clinical and social deficits than with neurocognitive deficits? *Psychopathology*, **35**, 280–288.

Power, A. (1974). *Conversations with James Joyce*. London: Millington.

Quillian, M.R. (1966). Semantic memory. Unpublished Doctoral Dissertation, Carnegie Institute of Technology. [Reprinted in part in *Semantic Information Processing*, ed. M. Minsky. Cambridge, MA: MIT Press, 1968.]

(1969). The Teachable Language Comprehender: a simulation program and theory of language. *Communications of the ACM*, **12**, 459–476.

Ragin, A.B. and Oltmanns, T.F. (1986). Lexical cohesion and formal thought disorder during and after psychotic episodes. *Journal of Abnormal Psychology*, **95**, 181–183.

Rapin, I. and Allen, D. (1987). Developmental language disorders: nosologic considerations. In *Neuropsychology of Language, Reading and Spelling*, ed. U. Kirk. New York: Academic Press.

Reed, J.L. (1970). Schizophrenic thought disorder: a review and hypothesis. *Comprehensive Psychiatry*, **11**, 403–432.

Reilly, F., Harrow, M., Tucker, G.J., Quinlan, D.M. and Siegel, A. (1975). Looseness of associations in acute schizophrenia. *British Journal of Psychiatry*, **127**, 240–246.

Robert, P.H., Lafont, V., Medicin, I., Berthet, L., Thauby, S., Baudu, C. and Darcourt, G. (1998). Clustering and switching strategies in verbal fluency tasks: comparison between schizophrenics and healthy adults. *Journal of the International Neuropsychological Society*, **4**, 539–546.

Roberts, M.A. and Schuham, A.I. (1974). Word associations of schizophrenics and alcoholics as a function of strength of associative distracter. *Journal of Abnormal Psychology*, **83**, 426–431.

Rochester, S.R. and Martin, J.R. (1979). *Crazy Talk: A Study of the Discourse of Schizophrenic Speakers*. New York: Plenum.

Rodin, E. and Schmaltz, S. (1984). The Bear-Fedio personality inventory and temporal lobe epilepsy. *Neurology*, **34**, 591–596.

Rodriguez-Ferrera, S., McCarthy, R.A. and McKenna, P.J. (2001). Language in schizophrenia and its relationship to formal thought disorder. *Psychological Medicine*, **31**, 197–205.

Rogers, D. (1985). The motor disorders of severe psychiatric illness: a conflict of paradigms. *British Journal of Psychiatry*, **147**, 221–232.

(1992). *Motor Disorder in Psychiatry*. Chicester: Wiley.

*Rossell, S.L., Shapleske, J. and David, A.S. (2000). Direct and indirect semantic priming with neutral and emotional words in schizophrenia: relationship to delusions. *Cognitive Neuropsychiatry*, **5**, 271–292.

Rowe, E.W. and Shean, G. (1997). Card-sort performance and syndromes of schizophrenia. *Genetic, Social, and Psychology Monographs*, **123**, 197–209.

Rumsey, J., Andreasen, N.C. and Rapoport, J. (1986). Thought, language, communication, and affective flattening in autistic adults. *Archives of General Psychiatry*, **43**, 771–777.

Salzinger, K., Portnoy, S. and Feldman, R.S. (1978). Communicability deficit in schizophrenia resulting from a more general deficit. In *Language and Cognition in Schizophrenia*, ed. S. Schwartz. Hillsdale, NJ: Lawrence Erlbaum.

Sarai, M. and Matsunaga, H. (1993). Symptom segregation in chronic schizophrenia: the significance of thought disorder. *Schizophrenia Research*, **10**, 159–163.

Sarfati, Y. and Hardy-Bayle, M.C. (1999a). How do people with schizophrenia explain the behaviour of others? A study of theory of mind and its relationship to thought and speech disorganization in schizophrenia. *Psychological Medicine*, **29**, 613–620.

Sarfati, Y., Hardy-Bayle, M.C., Brunet, E. and Widlocher, D. (1999b). Investigating theory of mind in schizophrenia: influence of verbalization in disorganized and non-disorganized patients. *Schizophrenia Research*, **37**, 183–190.

Saykin, A.J., Shtasel, D., Gur, R.E., Kester, D., Mozley, L.H., Stafiniak, P. and Gur, R. (1994). Neuropsychological deficits in neuroleptic naive patients with first-episode schizophrenia. *Archives of General Psychiatry*, **51**, 124–131.

Saykin, A.J., Gur, R.C., Gur, R.E., Mozley, P.D., Mozley, L.H., Resnick, S.M., Kester, B. and Stafiniak, P. (1991). Neuropsychological function in schizophrenia: selective impairment in memory and learning. *Archives of General Psychiatry*, **48**, 618–624.

Schwartz, S. (1982). Is there a schizophrenic language? *Behavioral and Brain Sciences*, **5**, 579–626.

Sedler, M.J. (1985). The legacy of Ewald Hecker: a new translation of 'die Hebephrenie'. *American Journal of Psychiatry*, **142**, 1265–1271.

Shallice, T. (1982). Specific impairments of planning. *Philosophical Transactions of the Royal Society of London, B*, **298**, 199–209.

(1998). *From Neuropsychology to Mental Structure.* Cambridge: Cambridge University Press.

Shallice, T. and Evans, M.E. (1978). The involvement of the frontal lobes in cognitive estimation. *Cortex*, **14**, 294–303.

Shallice, T., Burgess, P.W. and Frith, C.D. (1991). Can the neuropsychological case-study approach be applied to schizophrenia? *Psychological Medicine*, **21**, 661–673.

Shloss, C.L. (2003). *Lucia Joyce: To Dance in the Wake.* New York: Farrar, Strauss & Giroux.

Shorter, E. (1997). *A History of Psychiatry: From the Era of the Asylum to the Age of Prozac.* New York: Wiley.

Shtasel, D.L., Gur, R.E., Gallacher, F., Heimberg, C., Cannon, T. and Gur, R.C. (1992). Phenomenology and functioning in first-episode schizophrenia. *Schizophrenia Bulletin*, **18**, 449–461.

Siegel, A., Harrow, M., Reilly, F. and Tucker, G.J. (1976). Loose associations and disordered speech patterns in chronic schizophrenia. *Journal of Nervous and Mental Disease*, **162**, 105–112.

Simmons, J.Q. and Baltaxe, C. (1975). Language patterns of adolescent autistics. *Journal of Autism and Childhood Schizophrenia*, **5**, 333–351.

Smith, D.A., Mar, C.M. and Turoff, B.K. (1998). The structure of schizophrenic symptoms: a meta-analytic confirmatory factor analysis. *Schizophrenia Research*, **31**, 57–70.

Snodgrass, J.G. and Vanderwart, M. (1980). A standardised set of 260 pictures: norms for name agreement. *Journal of Experimental Psychology: General*, **6**, 174–215.

Snowden, J.S., Goulding, P.J. and Neary, D. (1989). Semantic dementia. a form of circumscribed cerebral atrophy. *Behavioural Neurology*, **2**, 167–182.

Snowden, J.S., Neary, D. and Mann, D.M.A. (1996). *Fronto-Temporal Lobar Degeneration: Fronto-Temporal Dementia, Progressive Aphasia, Semantic Dementia.* New York: Churchill Livingstone.

*Spitzer, M., Braun, U., Hermle, L. and Maier, S. (1993). Associative semantic network dysfunction in thought-disordered schizophrenic patients: direct evidence from indirect semantic priming. *Biological Psychiatry*, **34**, 864–877.

* Spitzer, M., Weisbrod, M., Winkler, S. and Maier, S. (1997). Ereigniskorrelierte Potentiale bei semantischen Sprachverarbeitungsprozessen schizophrener Patienten. *Nervenarzt*, **68**, 212–225.

* Spitzer, M., Weisker, I., Winter, M., Maier, S., Hermle, L. and Maher, B.A. (1994). Semantic and phonological priming in schizophrenia. *Journal of Abnormal Psychology*, **103**, 485–494.

Strauss, M.E. (1975). Strong meaning-response bias in schizophrenia. *Journal of Abnormal Psychology*, **84**, 295–298.

Strauss, J.S., Carpenter, W.T. and Bartko, J.J. (1974). An approach to the diagnosis and understanding of schizophrenia: III. Speculations on the processes that underlie schizophrenic symptoms and signs. *Schizophrenia Bulletin*, **1**, 61–69.

Stuart, G.W., Pantelis, C., Klimides, S. and Minas, I.H. (1999). The three-syndrome model of schizophrenia: meta-analysis of an artifact. *Schizophrenia Research*, **39**, 233–242.

* Surgaladze, S., Rossell, S., Rabe-Hesketh, S. and David, A.S. (2002). Cross-modal semantic priming in schizophrenia. *Journal of the International Neuropsychological Society*, **8**, 884–892.

Tabares, R., Sanjuan, J., Gomez-Beneyto, M. and Leal, C. (2000). Correlates of symptom dimensions in schizophrenia obtained with the Spanish version of the Manchester Scale. *Psychopathology*, **33**, 259–264.

Tamlyn, D. McKenna, P.J., Mortimer, A.M., Lund, C.E., Hammond, S. and Baddeley, A.D. (1992). Memory impairment in schizophrenia: its extent, affiliations and neuropsychological character. *Psychological Medicine*, **22**, 101–115.

Tantam, D. (1991). Asperger syndrome in adulthood. In *Autism and Asperger Syndrome*, ed. U. Frith. Cambridge: Cambridge University Press.

Taylor, M.A. and Abrams, R. (1975). Acute mania: clinical and genetic study of responders and nonresponders to treatments. *Archives of General Psychiatry*, **32**, 863–865.

Taylor, M.A., Reed, R. and Berenbaum, S. (1994). Patterns of speech disorders in schizophrenia and mania. *Journal of Nervous and Mental Disease*, **182**, 319–326.

Tenyi, T., Herold, R., Szili, I.M. and Trixler, M. (2002). Schizophrenics show a violation in the decoding of violations of conversational implicatures. *Psychopathology*, **35**, 25–27

Thomas, J. (1995). *Meaning in Interaction: An Introduction to Pragmatics*. London: Longman.

Thomas, P., Kearney, G., Napier, E., Ellis, E., Leudar, I. and Johnston, M. (1996). The reliability and characteristics of the Brief Syntactic Analysis. *British Journal of Psychiatry*, **168**, 334–343.

Thomas, P., King, K. and Fraser, W.I. (1987). Positive and negative symptoms of schizophrenia and linguistic performance. *Acta Psychiatrica Scandinavica*, **76**, 144–151.

Thomas, P., King, K., Fraser, W.I. and Kendell, R.E. (1990). Linguistic performance in schizophrenia: a comparison of acute and chronic patients. *British Journal of Psychiatry*, **156**, 204–210.

Thompson, P.A. and Meltzer, H.Y. (1993). Positive, negative and disorganisation factors from the Schedule for Affective Disorders and Schizophrenia and the Present State Examination: a three-factor solution. *British Journal of Psychiatry*, **163**, 344–351.

Tow, P.M. (1955). *Personality Changes Following Frontal Leucotomy: A Clinical and Experimental Study of the Functions of the Frontal Lobes in Man*. Oxford: Oxford University Press.

Tulving, E. (1972). Episodic and semantic memory. In *Organization of Memory*, ed. E. Tulving and W. Donaldson. New York: Academic Press.

(1983). *Elements of Episodic Memory*. Oxford: Clarendon Press.

(1985). Memory and consciousness. *Canadian Psychology*, **26**, 1–11.

Tyler, L.K. (1992). *Spoken Language Comprehension: An Experimental Approach to Disordered and Normal Processing*. London: MIT Press.

Vásquez-Barquero, J.L., Lastra, I., Nunez, M.J.C., Castanedo, S.H. and Dunn, G. (1996). Patterns of positive and negative symptoms in first episode schizophrenia. *British Journal of Psychiatry*, **168**, 693–701.

Van der Does, A.J.W., Dingmans, P.M.A. J, Linszen, D.H., Nugter, M.A. and Scholte, W.F. (1993). Symptom dimensions and cognitive and social functioning in recent-onset schizophrenia. *Psychological Medicine*, **23**, 745–753.

*Vinogradov, S., Ober, B.A. and Shenaut, G.K. (1992). Semantic priming of word pronunciation and lexical decision in schizophrenia. *Schizophrenia Research*, **8**, 171–181.

von Domarus, E. (1944). The specific laws of logic in schizophrenia. In *Language and Thought in Schizophrenia*, ed. J.S. Kasanin. Berkeley/Los Angeles: University of California Press.

Warrington, E.K. (1975). The selective impairment of semantic memory. *Quarterly Journal of Experimental Psychology*, **27**, 635–657.

Waxman, S.G. and Geschwind, N. (1975). The interictal behavior syndrome of temporal lobe epilepsy. *Archives of General Psychiatry*, **32**, 1580–1586.

Weeks, D. and James, J. (1995). *Eccentrics*. London: Weidenfield & Nicholson.

Weeks, D.J. and Ward, K. (1988). *Eccentrics: The Scientific Investigation*. Stirling: Stirling University Press.

Weinberger, D.R., Berman, K.F. and Zec, R.F. (1986). Physiological dysfunction of dorsolateral prefrontal cortex in schizophrenia: I. Regional cerebral blood flow evidence. *Archives of General Psychiatry*, **43**, 114–124.

Weinstein, E.A. (1981). Behavioral aspects of jargonaphasia. In *Jargonaphasia*, ed. J.W. Brown. New York: Academic Press.

Weinstein, E.A. and Kahn, R.L. (1952). Non-aphasic misnaming (paraphasia) in organic brain disease. *Archives of Neurology and Psychiatry*, **67**, 72–79.

*Weisbrod, M., Maier, S., Harig, S., Himmelsbach, U. and Spitzer, M. (1998). Lateralised semantic and indirect semantic priming effects in people with schizophrenia. *British Journal of Psychiatry*, **172**, 142–146.

WHO (World Health Organization) (1973). Report of the International Pilot Study of Schizophrenia. World Health Organization, Geneva.

Wilson, B.A., Alderman, N., Burgess, P., Emslie, H. and Evans J. (1996). *Behavioural Assessment of the Dysexecutive Syndrome*, Bury St Edmunds, Suffolk: Thames Valley Test Company.

Wilson, M. (1993). DSM-III and the transformation of American psychiatry: a history. *American Journal of Psychiatry*, **150**, 399–410.

Wing, J.K. (1961). A simple and reliable subclassification of chronic schizophrenia. *Journal of Mental Science*, **107**, 862–875.

Wing, J.K., Birley, J.L.T., Cooper, J.E., Graham, P. and Isaacs, A.D. (1967). Reliability of a procedure for measuring and classifying 'Present Psychiatric State'. *British Journal of Psychiatry*, **113**, 499–515.

Wing, J.K. and Brown, G.W. (1970). *Institutionalism and Schizophrenia: A Comparative Study of Three Mental Hospitals, 1960–1968*. Cambridge: Cambridge University Press.

Wing, J.K., Cooper, J.E. and Sartorius, N. (1974). *The Measurement and Classification of Psychiatric Symptoms*. Cambridge: Cambridge University Press.

Wing, L. (1981). Asperger's syndrome: a clinical account. *Psychological Medicine*, **11**, 115–129. (1996). *The Autistic Spectrum: A Guide for Parents and Professionals*. London: Constable & Robinson.

Wing, L. and Attwood, A. (1987). Syndromes of autism and atypical development. In *Handbook of Autism and Pervasive Developmental Disorders*, ed. D.J. Cohen and A.M. Donnellan. Silver Spring, Maryland: Winston.

Woodward, T.S., Ruff, C.C., Thornton, A.E., Moritz, S. and Liddle, P.F. (2003). Methodological considerations regarding the association of Stroop and verbal fluency performance with the symptoms of schizophrenia. *Schizophrenia Research*, **61**, 207–214.

Wright, I.C., Rabe-Hesketh, S., Woodruff, P.W., David, A.S., Murray, R.M. and Bullmore E.T. (2000). Meta-analysis of regional brain volumes in schizophrenia. *American Journal of Psychiatry*, **157**, 16–25.

Wykes, T. (1981). Can the psychiatrist learn from the psycholinguist? Detecting coherence in the disordered speech of manics and schizophrenics. *Psychological Medicine*, **11**, 641–642.

Wykes, T. and Leff, J. (1982). Disordered speech: differences between manics and schizophrenics. *Brain and Language*, **15**, 117–124.

Yule, G. (1996). *Pragmatics*. Oxford: Oxford University Press.

Zaslow, R.W. (1950). A new approach to the problem of conceptual thinking in schizophrenia. *Journal of Consulting Psychology*, **14**, 335–339.

Index